9 MONTHS—
a Joyful Journey

9 MONTHS—
a Joyful Journey

MITALI

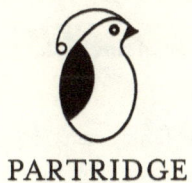

PARTRIDGE

To order additional copies of this book, contact
Partridge India
000 800 10062 62
orders.india@partridgepublishing.com

www.partridgepublishing.com/india

CONTENTS

Acknowledgements

Acknowledgement is not just a formality for me, but I really mean it from my heart. This book would not have been possible without the inspiration, encouragement, and support of my husband, Rajiv Mehta, who guided me throughout the process.

I would like to express my gratitude to the following:

My sons, Yagna and Jaival, and my family and friends who are my life chargers.

My colleague Jalpa Desai, a physiotherapist and a childbirth educator who is the continuous source of motivation and suggestions. She has also written the "Nutritional Baggage" chapter in the book and given her images of yoga poses.

My teachers Dr. C. G. Padole and Dr. Nilima Patel, who taught me the basics of physiotherapy.

Dr. Mugdha Wagh Shaan is my mentor, and under her guidance, I can see myself as a childbirth educator.

All the expecting mothers and future babies who become the continuous source of learning.

A very special thanks to Mrs. Shipra Narang and Mrs. Maithili Chintan Patel, who have given their yoga-posed photographs in the book.

Preface

Congratulations! So now you have planned to move or you already moved to a phase from a bold girlhood to a more mature and responsible motherhood. Actually we women are just wondrous. We play a variety of roles in one single life. We are the life giver, miracle creator, and magic maker. In every woman's life, especially, these 9 months of pregnancy is a lifetime experience to be cherished. Pregnancy is a time to relax, nurture, and support your body and mind as they undergo marvellous metamorphosis. We women have an amazing power to create, nourish, grow, and ultimately give birth to a new life. This 9-month long process of shaping and moulding that happens in your womb is an utmost crucial process as you prepare a very special world for your baby inside you.

Above all these, pregnancy is a time when soon-to-be mothers come up with so many questions and confusion, doubts and dilemma, and at some point of time, fear and anxiety too. Fear comes from ignorance. If you are not aware about what is going to happen next, fear and stress will definitely and automatically come. But once you get support of proper knowledge and awareness, there will be absolutely no doubts and anxiety. You are lucky enough that nowadays you have so many options and choices to get yourself well informed and thus prepare yourself for the upcoming challenges and a fearless childbirth. But sometimes, overload of information and advices you get from different sources make you more confused and apprehensive. Rather to make the things more complicated, many a times, it is better to just let it be and enjoy your pregnancy phases as they come.

Mindful-based pregnancy and birth is a new innovative concept evolved in the prenatal health. "Mindfulness" is a stress-busting and mood-lifting self-care program. It trains us to accept whatever is happening in the moment, without judging it good or bad and without striving to make things different. Pregnancy is a time when most of the women have a strong motivation to become the best person, especially the best mom they can be in a relatively short period of time. At this stage of life, you might be more open-minded and flexible, so it is a great time to explore a vast arena within you and surrounding you. Mindful pregnancy means accepting the experiences and changes of your mind and body with an affirmative and amiable approach. Live the present moment and enjoy your present status.

Whenever my expecting moms feel frustrated or emotionally disturbed, I always advise them to go for a small baby moon with their husbands. Always choose a natural location or resort for your baby moon. The quality time you spend with your husband will uplift your mood and rejuvenate the new you.

How this book has become my brainchild

When I was practising as a general physiotherapist, I came across many patients, especially my women patients, who actually inspire me to pursue my career in an obstetric physiotherapy. Most of my women patients with back pain or knee pain had their root of cause in their pregnancy. Due to lack of awareness and carelessness during pregnancy, their physical and emotional issues become chronic. Now as an ante-natal physiotherapist, I am working to create awareness about the importance of exercise, posture, and diet for a healthy pregnancy and fearless childbirth. Remember, woman's inner wisdom guides her through labour and childbirth. Childbirth education empowers women to make informed choices and assume responsibilities for their health and trust their insight.

The book *9 Months – A Joyful Journey* is a useful guide to all the expecting mothers. As we know, each pregnancy is unique and incomparable, you may not have the same symptoms and emotions like your sister and friend have in their pregnancy. Even you can differentiate the features, signs, or discomforts in your own pregnancies. So rather than discuss or analyse the pregnancy issues, you need to be aware and understand yourself physically, mentally, and spiritually. Accordingly, you can treat your body and mind for a healthy and happy trip towards motherhood. In this book, I have tried to put down all the facets of pregnancy every mom-to-be wants to and has to know. Women's confidence and ability to give birth naturally is either enhanced or diminished by the place of birth, her care provider, and above all, her own perception. So become aware that you have 9 months or 40 weeks or, say, 280 days in which to slowly emerge, nurture, grow, and reach to the climax of your pregnancy journey.

I wish you all the best. Stay safe, blessed, and have a joyful journey.

1

Concerns to Conceive

Once you have decided to start or expand your family, you might have to deal with many questions regarding how to start and succeed the first very important milestone, which lead to the path of a healthy pregnancy. Herein you have to work a little to make your dream *motherhood* more beautiful and not a nightmare. So take a few deep breaths and go through the following factors that need to be considered before planning for a baby.

FACTORS TO BE CONSIDERED

1 Check Yourself and Your Family Tree

a) Are you on some medication from a long time?

b) Do you or your spouse have history of diabetes, hypertension, cancer, thyroid, asthma, any infectious disease, or depression?

c) Is there any history of genetic disorders like muscular dystrophy, Down's syndrome, haemophilia, thalassemia, or sickle cell anaemia or any other disease in either side of the family? If any of the above answers is *Yes*, then consult your doctor and go for the pregnancy testing to rule out the carriers of these maladies. So accordingly you can be treated and/or vaccinated before you start trying to conceive.

If you have had any previous miscarriages, premature delivery, intrauterine growth retardation (IUGR), stillbirth, or previous pregnancy with complications, you have to discuss with your gynaecologist and keep her informed.

2   Diet Dose

You might have to struggle to conceive if you are overweight or underweight. If you do conceive, your weight problem may lead to pregnancy complications. Numerous studies have shown that specific changes to the diet can improve the fertility, prevent recurrent miscarriages, and thus support a healthy pregnancy. It is suggested to follow the instructions given below.

a) Stop drinking beverages containing caffeine or alcohol. Quit smoking. Studies have found that even occasional alcohol intake and smoking decreases the probabilities of conception. In pregnancy, consumption of alcohol and smoking lead to premature birth, stillbirth, or low birth weight. So STOP now.

b) Start taking multivitamins, especially folic acid, zinc, and iron (if anaemic) under the prescription of your doctor. Start at least 2–3 months before you plan to conceive. Taking folic acid helps prevent brain or spinal cord defects in the baby. So continue taking it throughout your pregnancy.

c) **Follow the fertility menu:** The natural fertility diet is based on the traditional diets that were followed in times when humans were most fertile, before the industrial foods. Apart from proteins and fibres, include a number of micronutrients (vitamin A, vitamin C, vitamin B_{12}, and vitamin D) and antioxidants too in your diet.

Eat organic food as much as possible, because pesticides affect your hormonal balance. Eat grains in their whole, natural form. Avoid processed and refined white foods and grains such as white bread, semolina pastas, and white rice. Instead go for the whole wheat/sprouted bread, wheat pasta, and brown rice. Prefer to eat a lot of plant protein such as beans, lentils, nuts, and tofu rather than animal protein.

Prefer to eat fresh and seasonal fruits and vegetables rather than tinned juices or processed food. Avoid oily, greasy, and spicy food. Stop eating the outside Chinese food, which contain high amount of monosodium glutamate (MSG), a very harmful chemical for our body.

Stop consuming skim milk and switch over to the whole milk. Take low-fat yoghurt every day.

Cooked spinach, broccoli, lettuce, and radish pods (mogri) are good sources of folic acid and iron.

Ginger, oyster, dark chocolates increase your libido.

Reduce the use of saturated fats, salt, and white sugar. Aim to drink 2 L of water every day.

Do not take high-dose painkillers and someone else's prescription drugs.

3 Environmental Factors

a) Stop alcohol and smoking. Even passive smoking is hazardous to both the mother and baby.

b) Avoid exposure to radiation. If X-ray is essential for other medical reasons, cover and protect your reproductive organs by a lead shield.

c) Air pollution, chemical substances like lead, mercury, or other heavy metals and pesticides are harmful and affect you and your partner's fertility rate. During pregnancy, all these environmental agents can reach to the baby via blood stream and harm the baby. So avoid going near the factories and more polluted areas.

d) Avoid hot tubs, saunas, and direct use of heating pads because continuously increasing body temperature can affect the ovulation process (release of egg). If you cannot ovulate, you cannot conceive.

4   Good Exercise Program

a) If you are involved in any kind of high-intensity or vigorous exercise program, dance, or sports, then stop it in order to conceive.

b) Yoga is the best exercise for your physical and mental health during your planning phase. It is very important to keep your body fit and energetic before you conceive. You have to strengthen and tone up your muscles for the challenging event of pregnancy and delivery.

Yoga for fertility: Certain yoga poses re-route the blood flow to reach the reproductive organs. Thus it provides more oxygen to these organs and makes them healthier. Yoga can detoxify your body, increase blood circulation, improve the immune system, reduce the stress level, and balance your hormonal status. This can help create a positive environment for a pregnancy, so it should be practiced by both partners. Always start your exercise or yoga after consulting your doctor and under the guidance of yoga expert or physiotherapist.

c) If you are overweight, first keep your weight under control as excess body fat can increase the amount of oestrogen in woman's body, which throws the fertile cycle out of balance. Exercise burns off the excess body fat and your hormone levels return to normal. But do not overdo, or it may give the reverse effect. Exercise may even improve your fertility if you are struggling to conceive because of polycystic ovarian disease (PCOD).

d) Regular exercise stimulates good hormones in the body, i.e., endorphin. It is our body's natural painkiller and mood elevator. So when you get pregnant, you can easily cope up with the mood swings that occur due to hormonal imbalance.

Yoga Positions

a) **Rhythmic rapid breathing (Kapalbhati Pranayama):** Prana is related to breathing and it is the universal principal of energy. The respiratory system is a bridge between the conscious and unconscious, voluntary and involuntary or body and mind. With the help of 'Pranayam', not only good habits of breathing are developed, but also control over mind is attained.

Sit comfortably in *Sukhasana* (cross-legged) or in half *Padmasana* position with your spine erect. Place your hands on the knees, palms facing the ceiling. Take a deep inhalation once, and as you exhale, pull your stomach in. Pull your navel back towards the spine. Initially you may keep your one hand on the stomach to feel the abdominal muscles' action. Your focus should be on exhalation, which is active and forceful as you are throwing your breath out. Your following inhalations should be automatic, passive, and shallow, and exhalations should be powerful. Take 30 such breaths at a time. Do 3–4 more rounds of Kapalbhati breathing. Always go at your own pace and stop if you feel dizzy.

Blood cells get purified with this Pranayam, and it further enhances the quality and quantity of reproductive cells. Once you get pregnant, stop doing this Pranayam till the 6–8 weeks postpartum.

b) **Inversion pose (Viparitakarni):** You must make sure to keep your stomach and bowels empty before doing this pose. Lie on your back against a wall. Now lift both your legs and hips up on the wall. You can use a prop like pillow, folded blanket, or bolster and slide the prop under your hips. You can also use your hands to support your hips. Do not strain your head and neck, and keep them in a neutral position. Soften your throat and your face. Hold this pose for 3–5 minutes with your normal breathing pace. Release and roll to any one side. Stay there for a few breaths and then sit up (Fig. 1.1).

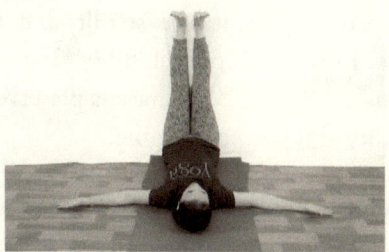

Avoid doing this pose during your periods and not advisable if you have some neck or back problems.

This pose involves contractions and relaxation of the anus and genitals and improves the flow of blood to the pelvic region. You can increase the chances of conception by remaining in the legs-up posture after sex. This asana has therapeutic values for anxiety, digestive problems, high/low blood pressure, headache, insomnia, depression, premenstrual syndrome, and menstrual cramps.

c) **Dhanurasana:** Lie on your stomach and keep both the legs together. Fold the legs slowly by bending the knees. Hold both the legs with your hands near the ankles. Breathe slowly in a normal pace and lift your head and look up. Stretch the legs a little further and arch your back to assume the posture of a bow. Remain there for a few seconds. You can increase the holding time with practice. Then release the legs, and lower them to the ground. Rest your head down and arm on your side. Take few relaxing breaths and repeat for 2–3 more times. This exercise stimulates all the endocrine glands, from the thyroid in the neck to the sex glands in the pelvic region. It cures sterility and impotence in men. In women, it is helpful in all irregularities of menses. Overall, Dhanurasana preserves youth and vitality and postpones aging.

d) **Standing forward bends (Hastapadasana):** Stand erect in *Tadasana*. Inhale and raise your hands up over the head. Exhale and slowly bend forward touching the hands to the feet. Release your head completely without feeling any stress on the neck. Keep breathing and hold the pose for a few seconds.

Inhale and come up. Repeat for a few more times. This exercise will improve the blood supply to the pelvic region and nervous system. This bend helps relieve stress from the abdomen region and stretches all the important muscles of the back.

e) **Cobra pose (Bhujangasana):** Lie down on your stomach on a comfortable mat with your toes flat on the floor and your forehead resting on the mat. Now, place your palms downward, under the shoulders. Keep your elbows parallel and close to the torso. Inhale and slowly lift your head, chest, and upper abdomen while keeping your navel on the floor. Now, straighten your hands from the elbow, and with the support of your hands, pull your torso back and off the floor. Ensure that there is equal pressure on both your palms. Continue to breathe gently. Hold the pose for few more breaths (Fig. 1.2).

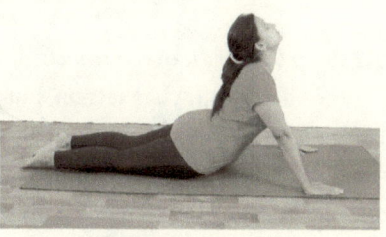

This exercise opens up the chest and strengthens the core body. It reduces your fatigue and stress and improves body blood circulation. Most importantly in females, this asana promotes a regular menstrual cycle. Once you get pregnant, stop doing this asana.

f) **Ashwini Mudra:** Sit in any comfortable meditation asana like *Padmasana, half Padamsana (Siddhasana), Vajrasana, Sukhasana* (cross-legged) or lie down on your back with knees bent and feet on the floor. Close your eyes and relax the whole body. Now bring your complete focus to the anus. Contract/pull the sphincter muscles of the anus for a few seconds and then relax them. Repeat this practice for as long as possible. Contraction and relaxation should be performed very smoothly and rhythmically. Gradually you can increase the holding time and make your contractions more efficient.

It is beneficial for genitals, prostate gland in male, and weak sex. This asana stimulates the abdomen and pelvic area including the reproductive organs and can improve your sexual health. It also has good effects on the uterus in women. You can continue this exercise throughout your pregnancy for the easy childbirth.

g) **Yogic sleep (Savasana):** *Savasana* might look like a nap at the end of your yoga session, but actually it's a difficult asana and you might struggle to be relaxed in the pose. Just lie down on your back. Hands are slightly away from the body and palms facing the ceiling. Your legs are slightly apart from each other and roll them outward. Close your eyes and focus on your breathing. Try to release tension from each and every part of your body and relax your mind too. Stay in *Savasana* for 15–20 minutes.

The physiological benefits of deep relaxation are decrease in the heart rate, blood pressure, muscle tension and anxiety, and increase energy level, concentration, and general productivity. You will get total relaxation (physical, mental, and emotional). This posture leaves you in a state of rejuvenation.

Any asana means to stay in position firmly with ease. The purpose of Yogasanas or any physical posture is to use the body to gain physical as well as mental health.

5 Preparations for Fathers

a) Although you are not going to carry a baby (until after delivery), you too have to actively participate and make a vital contribution in the process.

b) Cut down or better quit drinking habit. Quit smoking. Both alcohol and smoking reduce the sperm counts and lead to poor pregnancy outcome. If required, start taking multivitamin or male fertility supplement.

c) Healthy eating habits will give you the positive results because the better your nutrition, the healthier your sperms and more chances to conceive. Foods that are high in zinc like eggs, mushroom, whole grain cereals, selenium could increase your fertility. Eat variety of healthy foods, including plenty of fruits and vegetables which are rich sources of antioxidants.

d) It is also important to keep your body mass index (BMI) normal. So you need to exercise regularly and stay fit. Regular exercise is associated with an increased male fertility and virility.

e) You also have to avoid hot baths, saunas and electric blankets, tight and snug clothing, synthetic pants, and undergarments because if testicles become heated, sperm production will be impaired. For the same reason, do not put your laptop on your lap for longer time. Use boxer shorts rather than the tight briefs. Even cycling can cause a lot of friction and jostling, which increase the temperature of testicles.

f) Be relaxed and happy. Do not bring your job tension at home, because stress affects your libido, your testosterone level, and sperm production.

6 Follow Some Garbha Sanskar Tips

a) Garbha Sanskar is a Sanskrit word, which means 'Education in the womb'.

b) We know, in the Indian ancient times, the kings like Dasharatha and Drupad had performed sacred Yagna (sacrifice) to get divine child. Even we see birds and animals have their specific breeding season according to the nature's law. But we humans do not think about the healthy pre-pregnancy planning. We usually don't take in consideration the effect of our mental and emotional status during the pre-conception period. And then we complain about our children becoming more erratic, bizarre, and aberrant. So now if you have decided to get a healthy pregnancy and a dream child, both the parent has to change the lifestyle to some extent.

c) Stop late-night parties. Stop watching horror and action movies and daily soaps.

d) Take some time from your routine for yoga, prayers, and meditation. The term yoga has been derived from the Sanskrit word 'Yuj'. Yuj means joining. In the traditional terminology, yoga is the connection of the individual self with the universal self. According to 'Patanjali' (the Father of Modern Yoga), 'Yoga is a conscious process of gaining mastery over mind'. Regular practice of 'Ashtang yoga', improves your fitness and concentration, gives control of your emotions and temper, calms and disciplines the mind, and promotes contentment and a happier attitude.

e) Read some religious books and listen soft melodious music or chants. This produces positive vibrations in your home. Your mind and heart becomes more pure and lucid.

f) If possible, stop eating non-vegetarian foods, and turn to be purely vegetarian. Non-vegetarian food contains more parasites, fat, and bad toxins than the vegetarian food. In contrast to vegetarian foods, non-vegetarian food harms concentration levels and also increases anger and lust. Vegetarian foods considered to be 'Satvik' in nature. Satvik means ability to imbibe noble qualities such as peacefulness, concentration, love, and optimism in mind.

KNOW YOUR BODY

Pregnancy begins with the conception—beginning of a new life—and culminates with the birth of a baby. To understand this whole complicated process, which converts a single cell into a small human being, you need to have an idea about female body (Fig. 1.3).

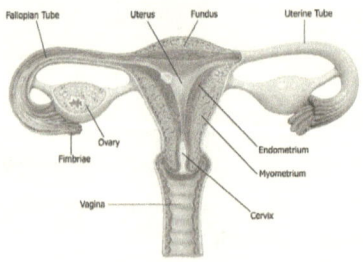

1. **Uterus:** It is a pear-shaped muscular organ in the lower abdomen region. The uterus consists of a body, upper broad fundus, and the lower neck or cervix. In the non-pregnant woman, its weight is about 2 ounce (60 g) and size is 8 cm long, 5 cm wide, and 3 cm deep. It is comprised of 3 layers: the outer serosa, the muscular middle layer, and the inner endometrium. In pregnancy, the uterus gradually increases 11 times to accommodate a fully developed baby.

   Sometimes the uterus passes downwards into vagina, the condition is called prolapsed uterus. It is caused by weakening of various supports of the uterus. So it is very important to strengthen the pelvic floor muscles, which support the uterus.

2. **Cervix:** The narrow lower part of uterus is called cervix or mouth of the womb. If you insert a finger into the vagina, you can touch your cervix as it protrudes into the vagina. It feels like a dimpled chin or nose tip. The entrance into the uterus through the cervix is very small and is called the cervical or internal OS.

3. **Vagina:** It is the outer opening through which the menstrual flow passes and through which your baby will be born. Vaginal opening is between the urethral opening and the anus. Several organs within the pelvis can be examined by the fingers introduced into the vagina. This is called per vaginal (PV) examination.

    Bimanual examination (with one hand on abdomen and 2 fingers of other hand in the vagina) helps in the assessment of the size and position of uterus, enlargement of ovaries and tube. Vagina is made up of elastic folds, which expands during childbirth.

4. **Ovaries:** There are two ovaries placed on either side of the uterus. Their size and shape is like an almond. Ovaries produce female hormones oestrogen and progesterone. They also produce and discharge ovum (eggs) every month. The process is called ovulation.

All women are born with about 1 million eggs in their two ovaries. You will release only 400 of them in your lifetime that too between your menarche (first period) to menopause.

5. **Fallopian tubes:** They are also called uterine tubes. They connect from ovaries to uterus on either side. They are about 10 cm long. They convey ovum from ovaries to uterus. Ovum is fertilized by the sperm, which travels from vagina through cervix into the uterus and from uterus to fallopian tube. Thus fertilization usually occurs in the last part of the tube.

Sometimes fertilized ovum instead of reaching to uterus, adhere to the walls of uterine tube, and start developing there. This condition is called as the tubal pregnancy or ectopic pregnancy. In such cases, you need to terminate it.

6. **Breasts:** The breasts are the specialized organs of the female body containing mammary glands, milk ducts, and fat tissues. In each breast, there are almost 15–20 lobes of mammary glands present, which become active during pregnancy. Each of these lobes is made up of many smaller lobules, which produce milk in the nursing women. Both the lobes and lobules are connected by milk ducts, which act as stems or tubes to carry milk to the nipple.

Nipple is the conical projection at the centre of the breast. The skin surrounding the nipple is highly pigmented and forms a circular area called areola. This becomes enlarged during pregnancy and lactation (breastfeeding phase). Oily secretion from its sebaceous glands lubricates the nipple and areola and thus prevents them from cracking during lactation.

After you stop using birth control, the time taken to get pregnant varies from one woman to another, depending on your age, your menstrual cycle, health of sperm, and viability of ovum (egg).

Ovulation is your most fertile time. In a woman with the 28-day menstrual cycle, ovulation occurs on about the 14th day (consider first day of your period is the first day of your menstrual cycle). The average egg has a lifespan of about 12–24 hours after its release. If you have intercourse on the 13th, 14th, or 15th day of your cycle (1 day before ovulation to 1 day afterward), there are the highest chances for you to conceive. If your periods are not regular, you can use an ovulation predictor kit, which is just like a home pregnancy test. It will give you an idea when you are going to ovulate. If you have the 28-day cycle, start testing from day 11.

If you are not getting positive result despite actively trying, consult your doctor. With the help of sonography, you can get the exact ovulation (release of egg) time.

Fertilization: Conception or fertilization is truly one of the nature's miracles.

After ovulation, the ovum is picked up by the fimbriae (funnel-shaped end of the fallopian tube) and it gradually travels down the fallopian tube towards the uterus. If intercourse has taken place during this time, then one of the thousands of sperms deposited in the vagina travels up through the cervix, uterus, and finally reaches the fallopian tube and fertilize the ovum present there. This grand event is the beginning of a new human being. The genetic material of the father is added to that of the mother in fertilization. Immediately after fertilization, early cell division results in a solid ball of cell, which is called a 'morula'. This growth occurs within 96 hours after conception.

Then fertilized ovum reaches to the uterus after a few days' journey and gets established in the thickened lining of uterus called endometrium. Now, once your pregnancy is established, the production of hormones stops the process of ovulation, and as a result, the menstruation stops.

2

The Roller-Coaster Journey Begins

A missed period is the first and most obvious sign of conception. But few females keep having their periods for the first 3 months of pregnancy; however, the amount and duration of bleeding is much less. Other physical symptoms include tender and tingling breasts, fatigue, malaise, nausea, and increased urinary frequency.

It is always better to consult your doctor or take a home pregnancy test to confirm the pregnancy. The home pregnancy kit will give you an accurate result if done after a week of missed period, and make sure the urine sample you take is the first of the day. The presence of beta-human chorionic gonadotropin (HCG) will give you a positive result. HCG is also known as the pregnancy hormone.

Congratulations, if now you have confirmed your pregnancy as positive. You may not feel any difference physically yet, but your emotions may be thrilling. You will experience the roller-coaster ride of happiness, anxiety, excitement, fear, and joy throughout the coming magical nine months. At different stages of pregnancy, you will come across so many questions and doubts and you will turn to your mother, sister, or friends for the solutions. But the fact is, each pregnancy is unique in its own way. What your sister or friend has experienced in their pregnancy may not be the same episodes you might experience. Thereby, it is better you understand your body and your pregnancy and accordingly prepare yourself for the healthy pregnancy and childbirth.

So let's move on to the next step, which is finding out your expected due date (EDD). Ovulation usually occurs between 12 and 16 days after the first day of your last period. So conception must have occurred during this time only. You will be considered 4 weeks pregnant when you missed your first period. That means in the first month of pregnancy, you did not know that you are pregnant. When you come to know about your pregnancy, it would be already a month.

You can calculate your due date by adding 9 months and 7 days to the first day of your last period, or you can subtract 3 months and then add 7 days to your last period date. This is accurate for only those women who have their regular cycle of 28 days. The other important source to get an EDD is an early ultrasound.

Above all these, records say that only 5% babies are actually born on their due date. A normal pregnancy can last anywhere from 38 to 42 weeks.

First Milestone (1ˢᵗ Trimester) Development

The period of first 3 months of pregnancy is called the 1ˢᵗ trimester. This is a little crucial period. As you become pregnant, hormonal levels of oestrogen and progesterone in the body suddenly increase, so you may feel a lot of physical and emotional changes in your body. By the end of the 3ʳᵈ month, your body is accustomed with the hormones and your pregnancy becomes stable.

Month 1 (Weeks 1–4)

At this stage, you are unaware about your pregnancy. During week 3, the fertilized egg cell travels through the fallopian tube and gets implanted in the uterus. Then it starts to grow by cell division and forms into a small ball-shaped, fluid-filled mass of cells called the 'blastocyte'. This further divides into two parts: the outer half will turn into a disc-shaped organ called *placenta*, and the inner half becomes the *embryo* (foetus).

Your physical symptoms are the same as what you feel during your periods.

- Your breasts become heavy and sore. Tenderness and tingling sensations may be felt.

- You feel more irritable and tired than before without any extra exertion.

What's Going On in Your Womb

- At this stage, baby is like a tiny tadpole or seahorse having a tail, not resembling a human baby. Its size is smaller than a grain of rice.
- In the last 2 weeks of the first month, neural tube develops, which eventually becomes baby's brain and spinal cord.
- Apart from this, heart, digestive system, sensory organs, arm and leg buds begin to form.
- Eyes and ears start appearing.

Month 2 (Weeks 5–8)

- Although you cannot see your internal changes, your uterus has started to swell and becomes the size of a small orange. More blood flow is being directed to the uterus. Your cervix becomes soft.
- Morning sickness and unpleasant smell may cause nausea and vomiting.
- Pregnancy hormone human chorionic gonadotropin (HCG) is at the peak level in month 2.
- Facial skin becomes smoother or prone to acne and pimples. Your increased

metabolism will dilate your blood vessels and may lead to hot flushes and red cheeks.

- High hormonal levels may produce mood swings.
- Physical changes include weight gain, softening of gums, and slightly swollen thyroid glands.
- Food aversion and cravings are very common at this stage. Excess salivation may occur.

Baby's Development

- Baby is taking oxygen via developing placenta. Amniotic sac (bag of water) is also developing in which the baby will be protected and growing for next 7–8 months.
- Baby is approximately 3 cm (1 inch) long and weighs around 8-9 g.
- Limbs have formed. At the tip of limbs, tiny fingers and toes begin to form.
- Upper lip and tip of nose are seen on the face. External ear structures are forming.
- The eyes are wide apart on the sides of head. Eyelids begin to form.
- The complete body plan is laid out, and for the next 6 months, continuous cell division and growth will occur on that plan.
- Tail disappears and he/she looks more like a baby than it was at last month.

- Brain is developing. Embryonic heart is developed and danger of any congenital abnormality can be ruled out. At this stage, his heart is beating 160–170 times per minute (more than twice as fast as that of an adult).

Month 3 (Weeks 9–12)

- The growing womb starts rising out of the pelvis, and it can first be felt in the lower abdomen. The size of the uterus is now 10 cm.
- Your heartbeats increase to cope with the increased volume of blood circulation in your body.
- So mother feels much warmer than usual and tends to sweat more. Drink lots of water/liquids.
- Occasional headache and dizziness occur.
- Fatigue, lack of energy, and sleepiness are the common symptoms at this stage.

What's the Baby Doing in the Womb

- Baby's head is growing rapidly. Face is well formed. At this stage, head is half the size of entire foetus.
- Baby's appearance is becoming more refined. Ears move to the sides of the head. Eyes become closure.
- Soft fingernails start to develop.

- Fine hair growth all over the body.
- At the end of the 3rd month, baby is almost 3.5 inches long, the size of a peach fruit.
- Baby can suck thumb. It can swallow and yawn too.
- For the first few months, the placenta produces amniotic fluid. As the kidney begins to function, baby swallows this amniotic fluid and passes out as saline-like urine, which again contributes to amniotic fluid. This fluid keeps the baby safely cushioned inside the amniotic sac (also called membrane or bag of water). Amniotic fluid contains a variety of substances like glucose, fructose, protein, urea, lactic acid, citric acid, salt, amino acid, and fatty acids. This fluid is also absorbed through the foetal tissues and skin.
- Baby's umbilical cord is fully formed about 50 cm long and 1.5 cm thick. Blood circulation has started through it.
- Prostate in male and ovaries in female begin to form. In boys, testes start producing testosterone.
- By the end of 3rd month, intestinal movements start.

I Trimester Tests

Now onward, on your every visit to the clinic, the doctor will do your physical check-up, which includes weight assessment, blood pressure check, breast and pelvic examination.

1. Blood test: In the 1st trimester, the blood test is done to check for the following:
    - Your blood type and Rh factor. If you are Rh-negative, an injection of Rh-immunoglobulin can be given to prevent sensitization.
    - Haemoglobin level to rule out anaemia. A timely diagnosis of anaemia in the initial stages of pregnancy would make it possible to restore the correct concentration of haemoglobin in the blood.
    - Immunity to rubella, chicken pox, HIV, hepatitis B, and other sexually transmitted diseases.
    - Blood sugar test to check for diabetes.

    A sample of urine will be taken at your first visit to confirm your pregnancy by measuring the HCG level (blood HCG test may be used). Urine test will help the doctor to know the presence of protein, sugar (glucose) level and pus cells, which indicate pre-eclampsia (pregnancy induced high BP), diabetes, and kidney infections, respectively.

2. Ultrasound:
    - In the 1st trimester, the foetus is very small, so a transvaginal sonography is to be done to get a better image of the baby. The probe is inserted into the vagina and it gives clearer images of the female pelvic

organs and developing pregnancy as the ultrasound probe is very closer to these structures. Transvaginal sonography is done with your bladder empty or partially filled. This procedure is usually painless, although some women may have mild discomforts while inserting the probe into vagina. If you keep your body relaxed and focused on the breathing, the procedure will be quite easy and smooth.

- If you are very uncomfortable with transvaginal sonography, you can opt for transabdominal after discussing with your sonographer. In the initial months, transabdominal sonography is done with the full bladder because the full bladder moves bowel out from the pelvis into the abdomen, so the doctor can very well visualize your pregnancy, uterus, and ovaries.

- Ultrasound sends high-frequency sound waves through your womb (uterus) that bounces off your baby's body. The echoes or reflected waves are turned into an image on the screen, and thus, you can see baby's movements and position.

After decades of clinical use and studies, there are no evidences that scan are harmful, rather they are very much beneficial. A 1st trimester ultrasound is performed for a number of reasons, including the following:

- To confirm the viability of pregnancy by detecting baby's heartbeat.

- To confirm the location of pregnancy (to rule out an ectopic pregnancy).
- To get the accurate due date.
- To assess the number of foetuses as well as the type of twins if there.
- To study the placenta and investigate any bleeding problem.
- To rule out the risk for chromosomal abnormality.

Performing ultrasound for sex determination is illegal and a punishable act. It should be discouraged.

Growing and Glowing Second Milestone (2nd Trimester)

Welcome to the amazing 2nd trimester. It is the middle 3 months of your pregnancy. Now you can share your good news with friends and relatives as the crucial period is over. Your pregnancy and your baby will become more real to you in 2nd trimester as you begin to feel movements and life within. These 3 months are typically characterised by quiet months. For most of the women, 2nd trimester is the most enjoyable and carefree period of pregnancy. The morning sickness and nausea subside and you regain your appetite and strength. In addition, the physical discomforts of the 3rd trimester have not started yet. As 2nd trimester is considered to be the safest, you can plan your baby moon at this stage. You can take a relaxing holiday with your husband in order to enjoy a final trip together before the many sleepless nights that usually accompany a newborn baby.

Month 4 (Weeks 13–16)

- Uterus is more expanding and is about the size of a small melon.
- Testing for spina bifida and Down's syndrome is done here by non-invasive blood test.
- Milk glands in breasts start functioning, which causes swelling and tenderness in breasts. Nipple and areola become dark due to hormone melanin. Increase blood flow to breasts makes your veins become more visible.

How's Your Baby

- The placenta is almost the same size as your baby. It is fully functioning and takes over the production of your pregnancy hormones.
- Very faint eyebrows and eyelashes are starting to appear. Although his/her eyes are still closed, he/she is becoming sensitive to light.
- Bone marrow development continues and bones are starting to harden.
- Arms can be bent from elbow and wrist. Baby is now able to make fist and he can kick too.
- Baby is about the size of your palm and approximately 6 inches long and weighs around 80–100 g.

- Baby's vocal cord and taste buds have developed.
- Head is growing to accommodate the developing brain and it is in better proportion to the body.
- He/she might even use umbilical cord as its first toy.

Month 5 (Weeks 17–20)

- Your weight gain is in specific areas like hips, buttocks, abdomen, and thighs. People can notice your pregnancy now.
- Most women will start feeling baby's movements. Initially the movements are like fluttering of a butterfly or popping bubbles in a fizzy drink, which is called 'quickening'.
- As the uterus grow, it puts more pressure on the lungs, stomach, and kidneys, which will result in shortness of breaths, indigestion, acidity, flatulence, and frequent urination.
- Increased blood volume in the body leads to soft and smooth skin, glossy hair, and sparkling eyes which is known as the pregnancy glow.

How Baby Is Growing

- Facial features become more distinct and clearer each day.

- Baby's skin secretes white waxy and cheesy substance called 'vernix' to protect fragile baby skin which is continuously immersed in amniotic fluid.
- You can hear your baby's heartbeats with Doppler device, which amplifies the sound. A normal foetal heart rate (FHR) is about 120–160 beats per minute.
- Baby's digestive system is now advancing to absorb sugar and water and it passes out solid matter to large bowel.
- At the end of the 5th month, baby is about 8–10 inches long, size of a large eggplant. Baby is approximately half the length of a full-term baby.
- Your baby has plenty of room and is constantly exercising by moving and changing position. Usually baby sleeps a lot as much as 18–20 hours.

Month 6 (Weeks 21–25)

- Back pain, bladder problem, sore feet, fatigue may affect you from this month. So start organising the things to make life as easy as possible.
- Baby movements can cause pain under your ribs, which can be relieved if you lie down on your one side especially on the left side.
- A dark brown line down the middle of your belly (called linea nigra) might appear due

to high oestrogen level in your body. A navel starts protruding out.

- As your tummy expands, the skin over will be stretched and lead to stretch marks, especially if your skin is dry and itchy. So keep your skin moisturized particularly the abdominal and breast skin. Skin pigmentation may occur on face and/or abdomen.

Baby's Growth

- Skin pigmentation makes baby's hands rosy pink in colour. Skin becomes papery and translucent. Many blood vessels are visible.
- Baby's movements are vigorous, especially when mother is resting.
- The face is almost complete. Eyebrows and eyelashes now develop.
- Head is still little larger than body, but limbs and torso are growing rapidly and lengthening the body.
- The brain and nervous system are developing rapidly. Baby will be able to pass messages of sensation to the brain and vice versa (receiving messages of control movement from brain to limbs).
- Rapid eye movements have been detected at this stage suggesting that your baby dreams. The eyelids are still closed, but the eyeballs can move from side to side.

- At the end of this month, baby is almost 14–15 inches long (length of a large banana) and approximately 1 kg weighs.

II Trimester Tests

1. The major test in this trimester is 3-D (three-dimensional) ultrasound. You can see your baby in even more depth and detail than a standard 2-D ultrasound. Your baby's facial features and gestures can be seen very clearly. Many doctors offer a CD or 3-D pictures of the baby to the parents. It's like a lifetime memory.

2. In the 2nd trimester sonography, doctor will analyse the foetal growth; examine for the suspected foetal anomalies like cleft lip, heart or other internal organ defect, or spinal cord issue; position of the placenta (to rule out placenta previa) and cervix; access amniotic fluid; and look for the birth defects.

Multiple Marker Tests

It is also called triple marker test or quad screen testing. It is a maternal blood screening to rule out any chromosomal defects (Down's syndrome) or neural tube defect (spina bifida), which leads to the deformity of brain or spinal cord. Down's syndrome is a very rare genetic condition associated with physical growth delays and mild to moderate intellectual disability. Spina bifida is a condition in which the spine of the child is not developed fully and so failed to protect the delicate spinal cord.

Two tetanus toxoid injections are to be given to you at an interval of one month in developing countries.

III MILESTONE (III TRIMESTER)

During the last 3 months, your baby will continue to enlarge as you continue to adapt. Some mothers may feel that enough is enough and long for the end of pregnancy and start of your new mothering role. You will be closely monitored in this trimester with more frequent visits to your doctor.

Month 7 (Weeks 26–30)

- Uterus is bigger and giving more pressure on the internal organs.
- Some female may experience breast discharge (colostrum) at this stage.
- You become slower, clumsier, and start getting baby brain (become more forgetful).
- At this stage, you might feel achiness in lower abdomen or along its sides, back pain, and sciatica, so maintain a good sitting and standing posture.
- Your cholesterol level may increase a little at this month, but it is not the cause of worry as it is the building block for various pregnancy hormones, especially progesterone, which is very important at this stage for breast development and uterus relaxation.

- Your heart is working harder than ever, pumping 6 L of blood around the body in a minute.
- Your abdominal skin becomes itchy and stretch marks start appearing.
- Constipation is a common complain during this time and, if ignored, may lead to haemorrhoids.
- Despite of all these, this is the month you can prepare for and enjoy your baby shower.

How's Your Baby Growing

- Baby can cry, cough, and hiccup. Hiccups are the result of baby's struggle to practice breathing movements and thus encouraging the lungs to develop.
- The baby can be able to taste the difference in the amniotic fluid. When you eat different foods, he/she might even react to it. Some babies respond to spicy food by hiccupping or by kicking.
- Baby becomes aware and interacts with his environment. He/she can respond to stimuli like pain, light, sound, and can open its eyes sometime.
- Fat begins to deposit under the skin, and thus smoothing out the previously wrinkled skin.
- Brain becomes more mature.

- Legally viable baby. If born at this month, baby can survive.
- At the end of 7th month, baby is about 16–18 inches long and weighs about 1.5 kg.

Month 8 (Weeks 31–35)

- Baby's head is down now, and its legs will kick your ribs. So sometimes you may feel discomforts and pain.
- Fluid retention may lead to oedema (swelling in hands and feet) and varicose veins. You find it difficult to wear your rings and old shoes.
- Your increasing body weight is responsible for your leg pains and cramps.
- You might struggle to get a comfortable position to sleep. Increase frequency of urination and baby's movements may disturb your good night's sleep.
- Some mothers may feel false contractions (Braxton Hicks contraction) at this stage. Although irregular and painless, these contractions are uncomfortable. They stop when you change your position or activity. If you start feeling contractions while you are lying down, it will end when you stand up and walk. Practice breathing through the contractions when you feel your abdomen gets hard and tighten.
- Your body works hard to provide oxygen and nutrients to your baby, so it's normal

to get fatigued easily. You may have trouble moving fast because it leads to shortness of breath.

- Emotionally you become more apprehensive about your labour and delivery, absentminded, or too excited.

Eagerly Awaiting Baby

- Your baby is able to hear and recognise the variety of sounds including mother's voice. Talk to your baby because the surrounding amniotic fluid will conduct the sound. Baby can hear mother's heartbeat and stomach rumbling too.
- Brown fat deposition occurs between its skin and muscles that will keep baby warm in the early days after birth.
- Lungs are still not fully developed.
- End of this month, baby is approximately 20 inches long and weighs more than 2 kg.
- Significant increase in baby's height and weight decreases its womb space, so baby's kicks may be less frequent and more forceful.
- Baby is most likely to be settled in head down position with the knees curled up into his/her chest (vertex or cephalic position). In case of breech position (buttocks or feet down instead of head), some practitioners may perform an external version to turn baby in head down position.

However, it works only in 30–40% of cases and the procedure is pretty painful. Since a decade, this practice had changed as a large international study concluded that C-section is safer for a breech baby than a normal delivery.

- The placenta reaches at its maturity. It is round and flat about 23 cm in diameter and 1–2 cm thick. In the last few weeks of pregnancy, the placenta is usually situated on the top half of the uterus.

Month 9 (Weeks 36–40)

- The baby will drop more down in the pelvis, so mother will feel lightning sensations as the pressure releases from the ribs and internal organs.
- Breathing and eating become easier.
- Now uterus and baby's head put more pressure on the bladder, so expect more urination at this month. Sometimes you may suffer from stress incontinence.
- You might feel thicker and whiter vaginal discharge.
- Pelvic discomfort and pain and swelling in your hands are common at this phase.
- Extra fatigue or sometimes you may feel extra energy (nesting instinct).
- Ready to start labour at any time. Keep your hospital bag packed and ready since your baby could arrive at any time.

Ready To Come, Baby

- Baby is settled in the birth position. His head starts to descend into the pelvis and get locked or engaged there. Its weight should reach nearly 3 kg.
- Lungs are now mature and ready to function on their own.
- Face has filled out and looks smooth and plump.
- Meconium (the first bowel movement of baby) has collected in the baby's intestine and will be discarded during or after the birth.
- Skull is firm, but not hard enough, and skull bones are not fused yet, so it can deform slightly when head is squeezing down the birth canal.
- Circumference of head and the abdomen are almost the same.

III Trimester Tests

- Urine test is to be done again to check any infection, presence of protein or sugar in the urine. Positive result indicates pre-eclampsia or gestational diabetes.
- Blood test to check haemoglobin level.
- In your 7th and 8th month, you will most likely have a check-up every 15 days. As the 9th month starts, doctor will call you on weekly visits until you deliver.

- Ultrasound is to be done to know which position the baby is lying—head down, breech, or transverse.
- Electronic foetal heart monitoring to see the baby's wellness.

Table 2.1 Weight gain distribution (According to the American Pregnancy Association)

Baby	3 kg
Placenta	500–700 g
Amniotic fluid volume	1 kg
Uterus	1 kg
Breast tissues	700–800 g
Blood volume	1–2 kg
Protein, fat, and other nutrients stored	2.5–3 kg
Tissue fluid	2 kg

Overall weight gain in 9 months should be around 12–13 kg. This is contributed by you, your baby, and the baby's little house. In the first 3 months, there may be no weight gain or a little weight loss in case you are vomiting a lot or you can gain up to 1 kg. In the 2nd trimester, the baby starts to grow and you gain around 6–7 kg. In the 3rd trimester, you put on around 5–6 kg. Some women find their weight holds steady or even drops off about 500 g to 1 kg in their 9th month.

3

Obstacles in Your Journey

The hormonal and physical changes of pregnancy result in significant changes in a woman's body. Your body at the end of pregnancy produces more oestrogens in one day than a non-pregnant woman produces in 3 years. Herein we will discuss some of the pregnancy's most common complaints (don't worry, as you may not have all) and their natural remedies like dietary changes, breathing, cleansing, and relaxing techniques as well as general information to relieve your stress. Since medication of any kind is usually not advisable during pregnancy, natural/home remedies, which can eliminate or minimise the problems, are most welcome.

COMMON DISCOMFORTS OF PREGNANCY AND THEIR REMEDIES

1. Morning Sickness

Approximately 70% pregnant women experience nausea and vomiting—the most unpleasant symptom of pregnancy in their 1st trimester. This can disturb you at any time of the day or may last for the whole day. In the morning, the symptoms are worse as you are NBM (nil by mouth-empty stomach) whole night. Morning sickness is because of decrease in the blood sugar level and due to sudden rise of pregnancy hormones, HCG, which is produced by the placenta.

Useful Tips

- Eat 5–6 small meals a day rather to eat more at a time. Eat before you get really hungry.
- Increase your protein and carbohydrate intake like wheat pasta, brown rice, and grains. Vitamin B_6 will be useful in nausea. Banana is a good source of B_6.
- Avoid highly acidic food like orange juice or lemon juice early in the morning. Basil, ginger tea, mint tea, peppermint, or sucking ice cube help in eliminating nausea.
- Avoid fatty and spicy food. Avoid strong smell and foods that trigger nausea.
- Keep some toasts or wheat biscuits near your bed. Eat them if you wake up in

the midnight or before getting up in the morning.

- Although carbonated drinks with caffeine are not advisable in pregnancy, having it occasionally is fine in case of nausea as it helps in reducing your sensations and gives soothing effect to your stomach.
- Relaxation techniques, aromatherapy, and fresh air will help you.
- Do not stop eating or drinking just because of nausea. You can use electrolytes drink as it contains minerals and sugar.

Some women may have to take anti-vomiting medicines under the prescription of doctor.

2. Bleeding Gums

Due to high level of oestrogens and progesterone hormones, gums become soft and swollen and thus catch infection easily. Deficiency of vitamin C can lead to bleeding gums. This is more common in the first or last weeks of pregnancy.

How To Come Out

- Maintain good oral health by brushing teeth after every meal. Floss your teeth daily. Rinse your mouth well. Use soft toothbrush and fluoride toothpaste.
- Massage your gums with your fingers. But make sure that your hands are clean.

- Take more calcium and vitamin C rich food. Limit your sugar intake as it promotes the tooth decay.
- See your dentist but avoid X-ray or any other radiation during pregnancy.
- If you smoke, quit it now.

3. Constipation

Increased levels of progesterone make your digestive system less efficient. The motility of GI tract decreases due to loss of tone. These are the main reasons of constipation during pregnancy. Sometimes taking iron tablets may make the symptoms worse.

Helpful Tips

- Take up to 2–3 L of water and/or liquids.
- Add dried fruits (raisin, figs, and apricots), variety of coloured vegetables, and salads in your daily diet. Guava, ripe papaya, and banana are helpful. Eat whole grain bread, cereals, and oats.
- Walk at least 20–30 minutes a day. Some exercises like knee-to-chest stretching will improve your digestion and general circulation.
- Abdominal (baby) breathing will stimulate the intestinal area and, thus, will be helpful in constipation.

- If iron tablets worsen your problem, stop it for a few days and continue taking folic acid.

4. Gas/Flatulence

Your body produces more progesterone to support the pregnancy. This hormone slows down your digestive process, which leads to the bloated feeling and subsequent gas. Weight of the growing baby puts pressure on the digestive tract, which further slows down the things. Gas may be a result of eating certain foods together. Keeping a food diary will help in discovering unfavourable food combination.

What To Do

- Avoid gas causing food like beans, sprouts, cauliflower, corns, onion, cabbage, apple, pear, cheese, fruit juices. Take 4–5 small meals a day.
- Avoid boiling the food for longer time.
- Chew food slowly and well.
- Walking or sitting in *Vajrasana* (Zen sitting) after a meal will help reducing this problem. Exercise like knee-to-chest position with side-to-side rock will help.
- Sit with your legs elevated. Doing so will take the pressure of baby off from your abdomen and thus your body can digest more easily.

5. Mood Swings / Stress

Pregnancy is assumed to be one of the happiest times in any woman's life, but many of the women may feel upset and sometimes feel like crying without any reason. Emotional changes are very common in the pregnancy and occur due to the powerful hormones of pregnancy. Iron or vitamin B deficiency can make you feel tired, irritable, and lead to depression.

Your changing body shape can disturb your self-image. You may have conflicting feelings. One moment you are thrilled at the prospect of having a baby, and the very next minute you may feel frustrated, angry, or terrified of your new responsibilities. New research shows that a moderate level of stress is actually good for the foetus. It tones up the foetus' nervous system and accelerates its development.

Help Yourself

- Breathing exercise and meditation/relaxation is the best way out. Anulom-vilom breathing (alternate nostril breathing) or baby breaths will help.
- Another way to beat stress is to exercise. Yoga and other Pilates exercises are beneficial to combat stress. During exercise, the body produces less of stress hormone cortisol and more of the calming neurotransmitter serotonin.
- Going for a walk, taking a relaxing massage, and listening to a soft music will

give your stress a break. Pamper yourself with pedicure and manicure.

- Create a positive environment around you. Keep yourself busy in some creative activities and develop your hobbies.
- Feel free to share your problems and feelings with your partner and friends rather than struggling with yourself.
- Take food containing more iron and vitamin B.
- Plan a mini vacation (baby moon) in your 2nd trimester, which will work as a stress buster.

6. Nasal Bleed / Stuffy Nose

Stuffy nose or nasal congestion is caused by inflamed and swollen mucus membrane of nose. Increase blood volume can cause some nasal capillaries (tiny blood vessels) to rupture. Lack of vitamin C is also a causative factor. High level of oestrogens and progesterone may lead to nasal bleed. Apart from these, cold, cough, infections, sinus problems, and allergies all may contribute to nasal congestion or stuffy nose.

Comfort Measures

- Avoid getting dehydrated as this can make nasal secretion thicker.
- Warm water sprays/drops to each nostril will moisten the nose and shrink the membrane.

- Apply nasal jelly or any lubricant like Vaseline.
- Increase vitamin C rich food like lemon, oranges, grapes, strawberries, tomatoes, cabbage, broccoli, etc.
- Apply pressure on either side of your nose and between the eyebrows with your fingers. Steady massage with firm pressure will be felt like drainage from the nose.
- Steam inhalation, humidifier will give you soothing effect and help you breathe better.
- Avoid strong smelling agents like paints, alcohol, petrol, cigarette, which can aggravate your symptoms.

7. Dizziness/Fainting

This mostly happens in the 1st trimester. Your heart begins to beat faster to pump more blood per minute throughout the body, especially to uterus, placenta, and breasts. Thus your blood pressure gradually decreases and your brain gets less blood. This ultimately results in dizziness. In the later months, your distended uterus puts more pressure on the major blood vessels and again dropping your BP. Anaemia (low haemoglobin) or low blood sugar may be the reason of dizziness.

Comfort Measures

- Do abdominal breathing with your legs elevated at 45° angle. Pace should be slow and deep.

- When you start feeling lightheaded, sit or lie down immediately. Always lie on your left side; this increases blood flow to heart and brain.

- Avoid strenuous activity and long hours' standing as it pools the blood in lower legs and blood does not return to the heart fast enough, which will reduce your BP and you feel like fainting.

- Take plenty of fluids, fruits, and iron-rich diet.

- Don't change position quickly and suddenly. Be slow in the movement. Take your time getting up from lying position— first turn to one side, sit up with your hand support, and then get up.

- See your doctor without delay if you faint or you have dizziness along with shortness of breath, blurred vision, headache, and vomiting.

8. Skin Changes

- Stretch marks, dry and itchy skin, acne-pimples are the common skin problems in pregnancy. Stretch marks are the reddish-pinkish visible lines on the skin, which appear as a result of tearing in the dermal layer of the skin due to the rapid stretching of abdominal skin. They form around the places where large amount of fat is stored, mainly on the breasts, abdomen, and thighs. Scratching the dry skin will lead to more stretch marks. According to the American Society of Dermatology, more than 80% women will get stretch marks after their 6th month of pregnancy.

- Powerful pregnancy hormones stimulate more hair growth on your scalp and body, but after delivery, this cycle reverses and your hair will start falling out. Nipple and surrounding areola become dark. Below umbilicus, a dark brown line appears which is called 'linea nigra'. This will fade up after baby's birth.

Home Remedies

- Although there is no proven treatment for stretch marks, some home remedies might be helpful in order to reduce them.
- For dry skin, use a mask made up of oatmeal and rose water. Make a paste with milk cream, turmeric, and gram flour mixture and apply on stretch marks.
- Calamine lotion and oil massage will be helpful. Even you can apply aloe vera, lemon juice, or egg white to decrease your skin problems. Use a cream or non-sticky oil (with a blend of rosemary, lavender, calendula), which contain vitamin A and E or collagen as they make your skin more supple and elastic.
- Take frequent showers with lukewarm water and drink plenty of water.
- Don't use the soap, which makes your skin drier. Apply moisturiser frequently.

- Avoid excessive scrubbing to the dark skin area. Use a sunscreen lotion containing vitamin B_6.
- Don't wear synthetic and too tight clothes. Wear loose, cotton clothes, which are skin friendly.

9. Back Pain

- Back pain is one of the most common side effects and frequent complains of pregnancy. Nearly every pregnant woman has experienced backache to some degree at any stage of their pregnancy. It occurs due to the poor posture. Your standing, sitting, and lying posture and walking with pelvic tilt significantly strain your back.
- Due to the uterus enlargement, the body's centre of gravity shifts forward. If your back muscles are weak, they will be pulled forward as your tummy expands and your spinal curve will increase at lumbar region leads to 'lumbar lordosis'. This will put uneven tension and pressure at your back muscles.
- Pregnancy hormones temporarily loosen your ligaments and make your back more vulnerable. Sometimes pressure of a baby on the spinal nerves leads to sharp or constant nagging ache.
- Emotional stress can cause muscle tension in the back. You may experience back spasm or increased pain in your back.

Prevention and Treatment

- Exercise can go a long way keeping your back and spine strong. Exercise keeps your muscles in good shape and strength and keeps your joints flexible, which support your back. Strengthening of core muscles is vital for your back. The core muscles include the pelvic floor muscles that support your undercarriage and those that circle your waist like a corset. Pilates exercises are fantastic for targeting the core. Exercise on a gym ball will engage your core and thus makes you more stable.

- Good back posture is the fundamental to general health and well-being. Your alignment affects your breathing, digestion, all the internal organs and muscles and ultimately leads to fatigue. Because of the poor posture in pregnancy, the back ligaments get overstretched and the pain may continue after delivery too.

- Make a habit to sleep on your side (preferably left), supported by number of pillows, to take any pressure off your bump. If you want to lie on your back, put a cushion under your knee, which tilt your pelvis and gives your spine relief. Use a firm mattress to support your back curve.

- Cold packs and back massage can help relieve your pain by stimulating circulation throughout the body.

- Avoid high-heeled shoes, which hamper your spinal curve. One-and-a-half-inch heel is perfect.

- Try to organise your things, especially in the kitchen, so that you don't have to bend from your back frequently. Try to arrange everything at your waist level.

- Avoid lifting heavy objects. Balance the weight between two hands when carrying shopping bags.
- When you have to pick things from the floor/ground, rather than curling your whole body forward, just bend from your knees.
- When you have to stand for a long time, keep a low stool near you. Rest one leg on the stool for a while, then change it and put another leg on stool. This way you can release the stress and tension from the lower back.
- Always sit with your back straight and well supported. While getting out of bed, first roll on to one side and then with your hand support slowly sit up. Like this you can protect your back.
- Counter pressure, double-hip squeeze, and knee press are good interventions for back pain. But you need your partner's help and he should be trained for these. These techniques are very much effective in back labour as well.
- **Counter pressure:** Either you lean forward on the wall (in standing) resting your head and both hands on the wall or you can sit on the reverse of armless chair, resting your head on the backrest of a chair. Now your partner will apply steady and firm pressure on your sacrum with the heel of his hand. For circular pressure, press firm and then make small, penetrating, and circular movements with the skin and underlying muscles. Deep pressure will release tension in the muscles.
- **Double-hip squeeze:** It is a form of pressure massage. You lean yourself forward either in

standing against a wall or in crawling position on your hands and knees (all fours position). Partner has to place his hands along your buttocks, fingers spreading outward and on the top of your hip bones. Now partner should rotate his hands inward with firm pressure using his palms. Palms should be in the fleshy circle of muscles, not on any bone. Do it 5–6 times and you will feel better.

- **Knee press:** You sit on a stable chair. Your back should be a few inches forward from the back of the chair. Your feet should completely touch the floor. If not, use one or two pillows under it to get them full support. The partner faces you while kneeling. His both hands are cupped over your knees. Now he will push your knees straight back (horizontal force). This will cause your back to go into a pelvic tilt and will relieve pressure off the back (Fig. 3.1).

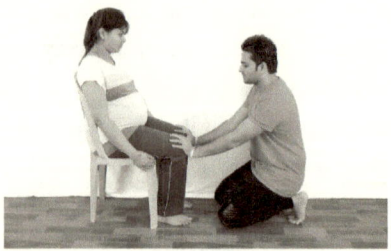

- **Consult your physiotherapist.** It's an investment in the future of your back. There are lists of yoga and exercises that are helpful in backache, but all should be done under a physiotherapist's guidance. Do these soothing exercises to keep your spine flexible.

- **Cat and camel:** On all fours position (crawling), gently pull your spine into a C shape (make your back convex) with head dropping down (chin to chest). Hold it for few seconds, and then compress it into a U shape (concave) with head up. Repeat this for 6–8 times. Your breathing should be natural and rhythmic. (Refer fig. 4.15.)

- **Chest opener:** In a standing position with legs slightly apart, hold your hands behind your back. Then bend forward while pulling your shoulder blades back. Make your back parallel to the floor and raise your head up. Hold it for 3–4 seconds and come back to starting position. Breathe normally and repeat the same.

- **Child pose:** In *Vajrasana*, kneel and sit back on your heels. Slowly bend forward so your forehead is on the floor. Then stretch your hands out in front of you, while pushing back into your heels. (Refer fig. 4.8.)

- **Pelvic rotation:** Stand straight with feet slightly apart. Place both the hands just below your waistline. Now rotate your pelvis in clockwise direction 10 times and then anti-clockwise. This will release the stress and relax the back muscles.

- **Bridging:** Lie on your back either on the firm mattress or on the yoga mat on the floor. Bend both knees so that feet are on the floor. Now lift your lower back and hips off the ground. Hold it for a few seconds and then release. Repeat for 8–10 times. Remember not to hold breaths in any exercise during pregnancy. (Refer fig. 4.9.)

10. Vaginal Discharge

Leucorrhoea is a medical term for thin, odourless, milky white vaginal discharge. Due to an increased hormonal level, glands in the cervix and vagina secrete more secretion to keep vagina clean and free from the infections. White discharge is normal, but if you have foul-smelling, yellowish, or greenish discharge along with itching and burning sensations in vulva (outside lips of the vagina) or if your vulva becomes red and swollen, you might have an infection. Don't ignore it and consult your doctor.

What To Do

- Always wear cotton panties and loose pants so that your skin breaths and absorbs sweating.
- Drink more water. Do more Kegel (pelvic floor) exercises.
- Clean and dry your vagina frequently to prevent the unpleasant odours.
- Wear pads or panty liners (never a tampon), which absorb the discharge and make you feel comfortable.

11. Fatigue

Fatigue or tiredness is very common in the initial and later months of pregnancy. This tends to be worse if it is your second or third pregnancy, because the expectant mother is unable to devote as much time to resting. In pregnancy, your metabolism is working harder, your heart is beating faster, and your belly and baby are growing bigger. Anaemia (low Hb level) may be the reason of fatigue. Haemoglobin level below 11g/100 mL considered low in pregnancy. If all of these combined with nausea, low BP, low blood sugar, you may feel completely drained out. In later months, your excess body weight and lack of sleep will make you fatigued.

Useful Tips

- Try to get an extra sleep at night and a short nap in the afternoon.
- Follow the diet rich in iron, protein, and vitamin C. Vegetables like mogri (radish pods), spinach, red cabbage, beet root are good source of iron. All sour fruits, tomatoes, broccoli contain lots of vitamin C. You get high protein from soya, cottage cheese, milk, and all the milk products.
- Take plenty of liquids in form of coconut water, juices, and soups.
- Avoid excessive amount of coffee, tea, and other stimulants as they are rich in tannins that impair the absorption of iron.
- Take out some time for exercise and a brisk walking, which will give you more energy, stamina, and improve your blood circulation.

12. Leg Cramps/Pain

Cramps are a sudden, sharp, and intermittent pain and contractions of calf muscles and feet. This may be due to incorrect calcium-magnesium level in the body. You can blame your hormonal changes and increased weight. Your growing uterus puts more pressure on the blood vessels and decreases the circulation in legs, which may lead to cramps. Whenever you are standing or walking, your leg muscles have to bear your body weight. If they are not strong enough, they feel strain and start aching.

Interventions

- Calf stretching exercise is the best remedy for cramps. Pumping action of feet will relieve your spasm.
- Rest with elevated legs; feet and calf massage, cold pack, or local heat will give you relief in pain.
- Have sufficient exposure to sunlight to meet vitamin D requirement.
- Eat a well-balanced diet that includes lots of calcium (yoghurt and milk products), magnesium (banana), and minerals (coconut water).
- Take a short walk daily, but don't try to stand for long periods and don't sit with your legs crossed.

13. Swelling in Hands and Feet

Swelling is due to the fluid retention which is a result of increased secretion of hormones (aldosterone). In pregnancy, your body is holding more fluid than normal, so the extra fluid tends to gather in distal parts of body. Pressure from the growing uterus on the blood vessels carrying blood from the lower body also causes fluid retention that result in oedema in legs and feet.

If you have numbness, tingling, and pain in your wrist and fingers, you may have a problem called carpal tunnel syndrome. Good news is that it will be relieved after delivery.

Comfort Measures

- Stop eating highly salted food like pickles, chips, canned and processed food.
- Have natural food with diuretics properties like cucumber, green tea, fenugreek seeds, parsley, garlic, and high-protein diet.
- Drink plenty of water and other liquids. Water is a natural diuretic, which helps to flush out all the toxins.
- Don't sit/stand in one position for a long time. Elevate your legs and feet while sitting. Avoid cross-leg sitting. Don't sit with weight such as another child on your legs (this hampers your circulation).
- Wear loose comfortable clothing. Tight clothing can slow down circulation and increase fluid retention. Wear comfortable flat shoes or open-toed sandals, which support the arches and prevent compression of the forefoot and toes. Pointed bellies are not at all advisable.
- Remove your fingers' and toes' rings. Pedicure will refresh your aching feet.

- Wrist and fingers, ankle and toes exercise will reduce your swelling.
- After a warm bath, roll your feet forward and backwards on a rolling pin, which will give you a massaging relief.

14. Varicose Veins

They are the enlarged, visible bluish veins in the legs. They mostly occur due to pressure on the large vein (inferior vena cava, which carries blood from legs to heart), which in turns increase pressure in the veins of the legs. Thus, they dilate to accommodate the extra blood.

Interventions

- Wear supports hose (compression stocking) if doctor suggests.
- Sit or lie down with your feet up higher than the heart.
- Change the positions frequently.
- Do not wear tight pants, socks, and belt.
- Do not sit in cross-legged position, not even on the chair.
- Take warm baths to soothe your legs.
- Apply an ice pack to relieve the swelling and discomfort.
- Foot and ankle exercise, walking, and swimming will help in the circulation.
- Avoid constipation as it worsens the symptoms.

- Try to control your weight gain as excess weight increases the pressure and exaggerates your problems.

15. Stress Incontinence

- Urinary incontinence is an uncontrollable peeing (leakage of urine), which can be embarrassing. But don't worry, it's normal and mostly temporary. This mostly creates problem in the last trimester. Baby's head is putting pressure on the bladder, which leads to the feeling of frequent urination. Sometimes you cannot pass urine completely in one time, but it may be in drops. It happens that you might feel urge to pass the urine, but you cannot. You might leak a little urine when you sneeze, cough, or laugh.
- In ladies, because of stress incontinence, urinary tract infection is very common. In female, the urine and stool holes are very near, so stool bacteria can easily enter the vagina. Urinary incontinence can be a sign of bladder infection.

Interventions

- Have lots of water and fibrous food.
- Cross your legs when you laugh or feel a sneeze or cough coming on.
- Strengthen your pelvic floor muscles. Kegel exercise is very important for pregnancy incontinence.
- Train your bladder just we do with the kids. Urinate every 30 minutes before you have the urge. Then gradually increase the time between pees.

- Alcohol, caffeine, acidic and spicy food irritate your bladder, so avoid it.

16. Insomnia (Lack of Sleep)

Sleep patterns change drastically in pregnancy, which is when the woman actually needs maximum comfort and a sound, peaceful sleep. With the increasing abdominal girth and overall size, mother finds it difficult to get a comfortable and her usual preferred position, especially in the last trimester. Back pain, shortness of breath, heartburn, frequent urination, and baby's movements are the additional factors causing sleep disturbance. Sometimes stress and vitamin B deficiency also lead to insomnia.

- Before going to bed, take a warm bath and have a glass of hot milk with honey.
- Wear comfortable clothes that allow your body to breathe easily.
- Yoga and deep breathing exercise, meditation with a soft music, and *Savasana* will relax your body and mind.
- Expecting mothers should rest and sleep in whatever position they are the most comfortable. If you are lying on your back, put a pillow below your knees so you won't get stretching in your spine and calf muscles.
- In some conditions, like if mother is suffering from pre-eclampsia (high BP in pregnancy), preterm labour, or other complications, the best position to sleep is side lying. It is said that 'left is right'

in pregnancy. Left is the best side to sleep as it relieves the pressure from the food pipe, liver, and major blood vessels of heart. Thus, it improves circulation and giving nutrient-packed blood an easier route from your heart to the placenta to nourish your baby. To get more comfort in side lying position, put a pillow between your legs and bend the upper leg slightly from the knee. During the whole night, you cannot sleep in one position only, so change your position according to your comfort. In certain cases, you can use specially designed 'body pillow' for maximum comfort in any position.

- Following the correct diet is also crucial as far as sound sleep is concerned. Eat right before you go to sleep. Avoid taking tea/coffee after evening. Avoid spicy and fried food. Cut down the level of fluid intake from late evening.

- In the last trimester, avoid lying on your back for a long time. There is a fear that heavy uterus may obstruct the aorta (the major blood vessel to the uterus).

WARNING SIGNS IN PREGNANCY

'Don't snooze the alarming signs in pregnancy'

Some symptoms in the pregnancy warrant immediate medical attention. Being aware of these danger signs can help you know when you may need special care.

1. **Abdominal pain:** Constipation and gas are unfortunately often part and parcel of pregnancy, which may lead to abdominal pain. As your baby and uterus are growing, you might feel a stretching kind of pain in the abdomen. It is usually occasional and gives you little discomfort. You could have pulled or stretched a ligament, which is common in pregnancy. But if you have severe, constant, or recurrent pain in your abdomen or tenderness in your lower tummy accompanied by backache, then don't ignore it and consult your doctor.

2. **Vaginal bleeding:** Bleeding in any phase of pregnancy is attention seeker. Some female may experience mild spotting in the 1st trimester as the embryo is being implanted in the uterus or due to the fluctuating hormonal levels. This is a normal sign, but if you have spotting or bleeding accompanied by sharp shooting kind of pain in the abdomen or lower back at any phase of pregnancy, immediately reach to your doctor.

   In the 2nd and 3rd trimesters, bleeding may be due to placenta previa. Placenta is a circular organ that develops in your uterus during pregnancy. It provides oxygen and nutrients to your baby via umbilical cord. Usually it attaches at the top or side of the uterus, but in some cases, placenta is at lower portion of the uterus and partially or completely covers the cervix. This condition is called low-lying placenta or 'placenta previa'. In most cases, it gradually moves up the uterus. In case if it does not, then you are supposed to go for a planned C-section.

3. **Urinary discomforts:** Increased frequency with small amounts, painful urination, blood-tinged urine, burning or itching sensations are the symptoms that indicate urinary infection.

4. **Neurological symptoms:** Severe headache, burning sensation in eyes, blurred vision, severe weakness, loss of balance, speech difficulty, whole body numbness, seeing flashlights or spots—all are considered dangers in pregnancy. Any of the listed symptoms is a call for emergency. Reach to your doctor without delay.

5. **Pre-eclampsia:** Pre-eclampsia means an increase in blood pressure and high level of protein in the urine. Primary symptoms of pre-eclampsia are sudden weight gain, excessive swelling of the feet and hands, and puffiness of the face (oedema). It affects several body organs and functions. Generally, reduction in the intake of salt and taking diuretics is sufficient to relieve it. If it is pregnancy-induced hypertension (PIH), then it will go once you deliver a baby.

6. **Vomiting:** First trimester nausea and vomiting (morning sickness) are considered normal and can be treated at home. However, if you have severe vomiting and diarrhoea lasting for more than 24 hours, it leads to dehydration. You might require hospitalisation and need intravenous fluids to replace lost salts and vitamins.

7. **Lack of kicking:** It is always advisable for the mother to use a foetal activity chart in the last trimester so you can track the record of baby's movements. Normally there are at least 6 moves per hour. However, if your baby suddenly moves less or does not move at all, it should be a reason

for concern. Sometimes it happens that if mother is quite active or busy someday, she may not notice the movements. In that situation, take a break from your work, have some juice rich in vitamin C (orange or lemon) with lots of sugar, and then lie down for a while. As the baby gets energy boost up, usually it will kick. But if you don't get any response from the baby, immediately notify your doctor.

8. **Preterm labour:** Labour that starts earlier than 36 weeks is considered as a premature or preterm labour. The symptoms can be any of the following:

- Four or more contractions per hour either with or without pain.
- Low back pain with pressure and heaviness in the pelvis.
- Menstrual-like cramps in the abdomen.
- Change in the vaginal discharge. It becomes reddish or brownish.
- Leaking fluid (rupture of amniotic sac).
- Woman in a preterm labour may be admitted in the hospital and given complete bed rest. If the cervix has not dilated significantly and the amniotic sac (bag of water) is intact, the pregnancy can probably be maintained to full term.

9. If you have fever more than 100°F and/or you combat fast or difficult breathing, then don't ignore it and consult your doctor.

4

Exercise for the Swift Journey

As we all know, people become very much aware about their body fitness. They regularly go to gym, do yogasanas, running, cycling, swimming, and so on. But when a lady becomes pregnant, she suddenly stops all these. Especially in India, your mother, mother-in-law, and grandmothers believe that pregnancy is a fragile and delicate stage. They want you to rest at home and not indulge in any kind of physical exercise. But this is a very wrong belief. In this chapter, we will see the benefits of exercise and the types of exercise you can enjoy throughout your 9 months.

BENEFITS OF EXERCISE

1. In pregnancy, as the body grows and mother gains weight, regular exercise helps in maintaining your health and comforts.

2. In pregnancy, your total blood volume increases from 30 to 60%. As a result, your heart has to pump 50% more blood per minute. The lungs are under pressure by growing uterus and your rib cage will widen up in order to compensate for this. A pregnant woman breathes much more air than a non-pregnant woman. Your digestive system is not as efficient due to the growing uterus.

   It should be obvious from these changes that controlled breathing and exercises during pregnancy are a must to adopt and cope up with the changes.

3. Exercise improves your respiration, circulation, and overall cardio-respiratory fitness.

4. The most noticeable physical change during pregnancy is seen in the musculoskeletal system. Growth of baby and uterus put more stress on your bones, muscles, and joints. So regular exercise tones up and strengthens the muscles affected by pregnancy including abdominal, lower back, pelvic floor, and lower limb muscles.

5. Exercise prevents the excessive accumulation of body fat. So being active helps you feel better about yourself and improve your odds of gaining unwanted weight. Thus, it gives you positive self-image.

6. It is scientifically proven that when you exercise, the body releases some chemicals called 'endorphins'.

Endorphin interacts with the brain receptors that reduces your perception of pain and triggers positive feelings in the body. Therefore, endorphins are the natural pain reliever of our body, which is found in higher amount in the exercising mothers.

7. Regular exercise will reduce your pregnancy discomforts like backache, constipation, leg oedema, cramps, insomnia (lack of sleep), etc.

8. Studies have found that exercise boosts up the level of 'serotonin', a brain chemical linked to mood, which puts you in a better spirit. It reduces your stress and helps to cope up with the mood swings.

9. The physical energy, endurance power, and mental focus gained through an exercise program will be effectively helpful in your labour and delivery. Childbirth is a life-changing experience, which requires more stamina, determination, and focus. Although prenatal exercise and physical fitness do not guarantee for normal and easy labour, but they definitely give mother more stamina to cope with a long, hard labour and more awareness to help work with the body during labour.

10. After delivery, many women come to us with complaints of flabby tummy and they are ready to do anything to get a slim body and flat tummy. So the good news is if you have maintained your strength, muscle tone, and good physical condition throughout your pregnancy, your body will bounce back quickly and easily after baby's birth. Your body's recovery rate will be fast, and the energy level, strength, and comeback in your pre-pregnant size will be motivation to others.

11. Physical exercise has also been shown to decrease the incidence of postpartum depression. During exercise, the body produces less of stress hormone called 'cortisol' and more of the calming neurotransmitter called 'serotonin'. Women who exercise regularly feel more accomplished, confident, and positive about life.

12. With the low-impact aerobics and Pilates exercises, the placental efficiency of exchange of oxygen–carbon dioxide and nutrients–waste products will increase. When you exercise, you are making your baby's cardiovascular capacity strong. Chances of baby becoming obese or diabetic in future are very less. Research shows that the babies of mothers who exercise regularly during their pregnancy are smarter and healthier.

13. According to the American College of Obstetrician and Gynaecologists, unless there are medical reasons, all pregnant women can and should exercise at least 30 minutes daily to obtain health benefits of exercise.

Contraindications or Warning Signs

Nowadays, more information and videos are available on internet and some enthusiastic mothers start doing exercise on their own. However, it is always advisable to do it under the guidance of a physiotherapist or childbirth educator. Even before starting any exercise program, consult your gynaecologist. Following are some complications or conditions in which you are not supposed to do exercise.

- Previous miscarriage

- Placenta previa (a condition where the placenta is adjacent to or blocks the cervix)
- Any heart or lung disease
- In case of twins or triplets
- Persistent vaginal bleeding
- History of preterm labour
- Incompetent cervix
- Intrauterine growth retardation
- High blood pressure (pre-eclampsia)
- Severe anaemia
- If you feel shortness of breath, headache, chest pain, severe back or pelvic pain, dizziness during or after exercise, then just stop doing exercise and consult your doctor.
- Avoid any exercise and sports that involve jumping, risk of falling, jerky movements, or sudden change in the direction.

TIPS AND GUIDELINES FOR SAFE AND EFFECTIVE EXERCISE

1. Wear loose and comfortable clothing. Do floor exercise on a comfortable foam mat or a carpet.
2. Deep breathing exercise should be done before, after, and in between the exercise session. Never hold your breath.
3. Always include warm-up and cool-down period after any stretching, strengthening, or light aerobics exercise.
4. Drink lots of water to prevent dehydration. Don't exercise in very hot and humid weather. Your basal metabolic rate (BMR – the energy you burn to stay

alive) is higher in pregnancy, so be careful not to get overheated.

5. Regular exercise sessions (at least 3 times a week – each session lasts for 30–40 minutes) are safer than intermittent burst of activities.

6. Vigorous exercise should not be continued for longer than 15 minutes.

7. It is essential that the women who are accustomed to a sedentary lifestyle should start with low-intensity physical activity such as walking, yoga, or static cycling. Always increase your activity level gradually according to your own individual tolerance capacity.

8. During pregnancy, the hormone relaxin makes your joints looser and more flexible in preparation for birth. Overextending your joints may cause injury. In stretching exercise, don't force your body to complete the range of motion (ROM). Your body is a warning alarm which gives you warning signals, don't ignore it and don't overdo.

I STAGE EXERCISE PROGRAM

The 1st trimester is said to be the delicate phase of pregnancy as you adopt to hormonal changes and your baby undergoes the most rapid and crucial early formation of the nervous system, so it is not advisable to indulge in any more strengthening, stretching, or aerobics exercise. The main aim of exercise in the 1st trimester is to nurture yourself with the slow movement accompanied by flow of your breath. Prepare your body for the postural and muscular changes that are going to occur in the coming months. Another benefit of 1st

stage exercise is to combat stress (mood swings) that occur at this phase due to sudden high hormonal level.

1. Abdominal Breathing Exercise

This is also called baby breathing or belly breathing. Sit cross-legged on the floor using a mat or any firm mattress. Close your eyes so that you can focus on your breathing. Place both hands on your abdomen and feel your baby inside. As your inhale, your tummy should rise (expand out) rather than your chest. There should not be any visible movement in the chest. While exhaling, your belly should fall in its normal position.

Use your imagination. Inhale imaging that air is going directly to your child through your navel. You can exhale either through your nose or through your mouth. This is a very important breathing exercise; try to practice it several times a day (Fig. 4.1). Baby breathing provides more oxygen to baby and at the 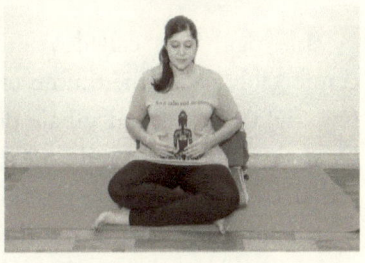 same time improves tone of your abdominal muscles.

2. Chest Expansion Breathing

It is also called 'diaphragmatic breathing'. If you are unable to sit cross-legged, keep your legs straight and take full support to your back (sit against the wall). Place both the hands just below your breasts on the side chest wall. Thumbs should face backwards and fingers forward. Close your eyes. Take one deep and slow inhalation with the feeling that your ribcage is expanding out and rising. Your spine is extending more and providing more oxygen to your body. Then exhale slowly with the feeling that your body is getting relaxed and loose. Repeat it again. You can exhale through your mouth to get more relaxation. Practice this breathing for at least 15 minutes. Remember, you don't have to hold the breaths in any kind of breathing exercise during pregnancy (Fig. 4.2). This kind of deep breathing will improve your lung functions and improve your mood and energy level.

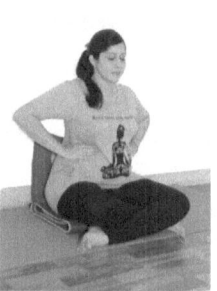

3. Alternate Nostril Breathing

In yoga, it is called 'Anulom-vilom pranayam'. Sit comfortably. With the thumb of your one hand, close one (say, right) nostril and inhale deeply through left nostril. Open the right nostril and close the left nostril to breathe out (exhale). Don't change the position and breathe in with right nostril only, then breathe out through left, again breathe in with left and breathe out through right, breathe in through right and so on. Keep your eyes closed during pranayam and feel your breaths. Practise it initially for 3–5 minutes and you can reach up to 10 minutes. You can change your hand if one is fatigued.

In pregnancy, this breathing is very useful to relieve stress and anxiety. It increases the oxygen supply throughout the body. In case of headache or insomnia (lack of sleep) in pregnancy, practice this pranayam in the evening or before sleep. You will surely get good result.

4. Neck Movements

In sitting or standing position, keep your body erect and shoulders relaxed. Slowly do upward and downward movements of neck. Stretch your neck as much you can in both the directions. Do 6–8 repetitions. Now, turn your head to right side and stretch up to the most available pain-free range of motion without turning your upper body. Hold it there for 2–3 seconds. Then turn towards the left extreme. Do these movements very slowly and swiftly without any jerks.

Lateral Neck Stretch

In the same position, tilt your head to one side without bending it forward, just like trying to touch your ear to the shoulder. However, remember not to raise your shoulder. Hold it for 2–3 seconds. You can apply a gentle pressure with your same sided hand to increase the stretch. Repeat this on the other side. These exercises are helpful in reducing the stiffness and any kind of pain in the neck. They also help in case of headache and insomnia.

5. Shoulder and Hand Exercises

Keep both your hands straight at the shoulder level, close your fingers and thumb (making fist), and open them. Do it for 10–15 times. Then do same movements with thumb pressing inside your fist. Maintain the same hand position, encircle your fist clockwise, and then anti-clockwise. Here you are getting rotational movement at wrist joint. Then, stretch your palms inside and out for a few times. Practice all these movements throughout your pregnancy and you will never complain the swelling or pain in the hands.

- **Elbow circles:** Bend your arms and place the palms on your shoulders with the fingers facing downward. Begin to make circles with your elbows as large as you can. Then reverse it and make large circles backwards. Do it for 8–10 times in each direction. Leave and relax your hands and take 1–2 deep breaths (Fig. 4.3).

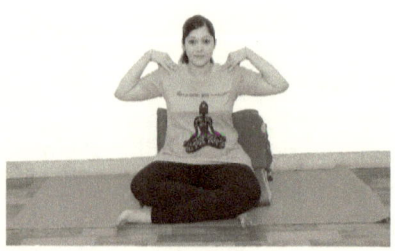

- **Shoulder shrugs:** Sitting or standing in an erect position, just raise both your shoulders up as if you are trying to touch your ears. Raise both the shoulders simultaneously and up to the same level. Hold it there for 2 seconds and then slowly down. Never do jerky movements, and when you put your shoulder down, there should not be any tension in your shoulder muscles. Repeat this for at least 10 times. You can incorporate breathing with shoulder shrugs. Inhale while you raise the shoulders up and exhale as you put them down.

All these above-mentioned exercises are highly recommended for the women who work at desk for long hours. Use it often during your work day.

- **Shoulder-rotator cuff stretching:** This is an easier modification of 'Cow head pose' (Gomukhasana). Do it in a cross-legged sitting position or in a Vajrasana. Raise your one hand (say, right arm) up and bend it from elbow, facing the palm in and try to bring the right hand to the centre of your back. Bend your left arm and bring it behind your back with palms facing out. Now try to bring both the hands as close as each other and touch them. Keep the top elbow high up in the air so it resembles a cow's horn. Hold this pose for 5–8 seconds. Keep your breathing at normal pace. Slowly separate the hands and repeat it on the other side with left hand up and right hand from below. Remember to keep your back straight and do not try to overstretch beyond your limits. You can use props like towel, belt or stick to complete the movement. This exercise opens up your chest and thoracic spine. It stretches the internal and external rotators of the shoulders.

6. Wall Lean

Usually we have a poor habit of shifting our head slightly forward especially in sitting posture, which may lead to shoulder and neck pain. Wall stand exercise focuses on the relationship to the shoulder girdle and head/neck position.

Stand with your back against a wall. Lean your head slightly backwards so that the back of the head touches the wall completely. Use a towel roll to cushion your head. Take 2 steps away from the wall, keeping only your head against the towel. Tilt your head slightly back so that head and your body should align in a straight line. Hold it for a minimum 20–25 seconds. Then slowly bring both the feet backwards one by one to come in a normal standing posture. Regular practise can help correcting the faulty posture.

In this position, you can press your back of head against the wall and feel the tension in your neck muscles. This is the static contraction of neck muscles. Press it for a few seconds and then release. Repeat it for 8–10 times. This strengthens your neck muscles.

All these neck and upper limb exercises will show their beneficial result even after delivery too. Mothers will never complain of neck and shoulder pain when they have to feed their babies frequently. You will never complain fatigue, tiredness, or numbness in the hands when you have to carry/ lift your baby for a longer time, as your muscles are now strong enough to bear the weight of your growing babies. You would not need pram, stroller, or carrycot anymore. You will love to carry your baby and increase the bond of love with each other.

7. Foot Exercise

In long sitting position on mat with your legs extended and knees straight, curl your toes inside and then extend up. Do it rhythmically and for about 20–25 times.

8. Ankle Stretching

In same position, stretch your feet up and towards the body so that you feel stretching in the calf muscles. Hold it for 3 seconds and then push your feet downward towards the floor. Do this for 10–15 times. Move your ankle and feet inside such that the soles of feet face each other and then move outside. Do it in a pain-free range and up to the moderate stretch. Do this 10 times.

Next, do circular movement of your ankle and feet in a clockwise direction and then anti-clockwise direction (10 times each side). These simple ankle-foot exercises work as a pumping action of leg, which will never allow the fluid retention in your feet and thus you will never experience oedema or swelling in the legs. Ankle stretching is the best exercise for cramps and leg pain.

9. Static Quadriceps

This is very simple exercise useful to protect your vulnerable knees as they have to bear your body's increased weight. In long sitting position, keep both the legs straight. Put small folded towel below your knees. Tighten your knees and press them downward. You can see and feel that your thigh muscles are working here. Hold it for 5 seconds and then release it. Repeat for at least 20–25 times on both the knees.

10. Pelvic Floor Exercise (Kegel Exercise, Ashwini Mudra)

Pelvic floor muscles are attached to the inside of pelvic bone and they act like cushion to support the internal vital abdominal and pelvic organs. During pregnancy, these muscles sag due to increased weight of uterus and relaxing effect of hormones.

Kegel exercise is very important to maintain the tone and improve circulation in the vaginal area. If the muscles are in good tone, it means they have good elasticity, so during delivery, they will stretch to allow childbirth and also come back to their original length postpartum. If you want easier, quicker, and comfortable delivery, learn to relax these muscles rather than tighten them during labour.

Kegel exercises should be continued after delivery as well. It is very important to maintain the strength and tone of these muscles so that you will never experience the problems of stress incontinence (leaking of urine while coughing, sneezing, or laughing).

How To Do

Contract or tighten the muscles of perineum (the area between vagina and anus) as if you are trying to stop the flow of urine. You will feel the tension and a slight lifting of pelvic floor. Initially just pull it and release. Gradually with the practice, you can hold the contractions for a few seconds. With the perfection, you try to hold it as tight as possible for a few more seconds. Imagine that everything is moving upward, floor by floor like a lift. Hold at each floor for 3 seconds. Make sure you are not tightening your buttocks and tummy. Do at least 8–10 contractions in one sitting and do several sittings in a day. Remember never perform pelvic floor exercise while you are passing urine as this may lead to a risk of developing a urine infection.

II and III STAGES EXERCISE PROGRAM

By the end of the 1st trimester, your pregnancy becomes established and stable. In the 2nd and 3rd trimesters, you experience internal and external physical changes in your body, which lead to more discomforts.

The main aim of exercise during 2nd trimester is to focus on building strength and stamina and improve/increase your vitality. Learn to expand your breathing capacity and agility, which help you to keep the right balance between activities and rest.

In the 3rd trimester, as you are practiced and adopted with I and II stage exercises, a slow and safe progression should be done towards stage III exercise. Use the power of breath to tone the deepest muscles is the advantage of **Pilates exercise**. Combination of movements to stretch and strengthen the whole body is what we call **'salute to baby'**. You can continue the 1st stage exercises in your 2nd and 3rd trimesters as well.

Floor Exercises in Sitting Position

Butterfly Exercise

- In yoga, this exercise is called 'Bhadrasana'. Sit with legs outstretched with soles of feet together and heels touching the perineum. Hold your feet together with the clasp of your hands. Here, knees are pointing outside. Now slowly press your knees towards the floor as low as you can. Do up and down movements of knees very swiftly and rhythmically. In next step, with the same legs position, slowly bend forward as you are trying to touch your head to your feet (Fig. 4.4).

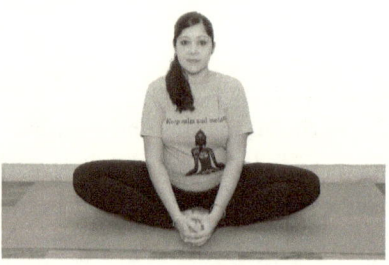

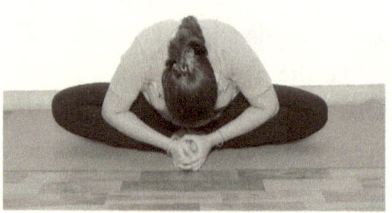

- The most important benefit of this exercise in pregnancy is that it stretches your inner thighs, groin, and opens up your hips. It strengthens your pelvic floor muscles, which is very important for an easy labour.

Vajrasana (Kneeling Position)

- Sit on your bent knees with a straight posture and upright spine. Your feet rest flat on the ground with soles turned upward. Place and support buttocks in the cavity thus formed. Remember to put equal weight on both the knees. If you feel pressure on your knees or pain in the knees, you can use pillow under your knees or between the thighs and legs. Hold this pose as long as you feel comfortable (Fig. 4.5).

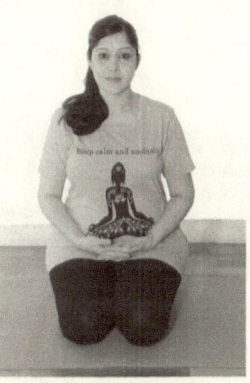

- Vajrasana is a good pose to do breathing exercise what we discussed earlier. Vajrasana is the only pose that can be done on a full stomach. In fact, it is advisable to sit in this pose after meal as it increases the blood flow towards pelvic area and stomach and thus facilitate digestion.
- Vajrasana is also good for your thighs, legs, hips, back, and ankles.
- Avoid doing this asana in case of any leg or knee injury.

Parvatasana (Mountain Pose)

- Sit in a sukhasana (cross-legged) or in a vajrasana
  position. Stretch your arms sideways and slowly
  bring them over your head with a deep and slow
  inhalation. Let your palms touch each other. Stretch
  your hands well without bending your elbows.
  Spine should be erect. Hold it for a few seconds,
  then bring hands down with exhalation (Fig. 4.6).

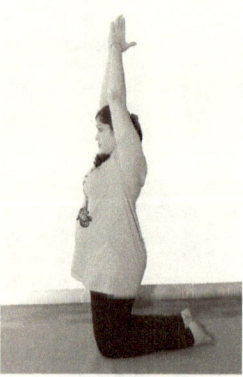

- This exercise stretches the spine and thus relieves
  back pain and corrects any postural defects. This
  stretching pose reduces extra fat from your back and
  waist. The chest and trunk muscles get strengthened.
  It provides more oxygenation to your body.

Leg Stretching to the Sides

- Sit on your mat with legs wide apart in an open V
  position. Keep your spine erect. Clasp your hands,
  and with one inhalation, bring them above your
  head. Hands should be stretched from elbow and

shoulders. Now bring the right hand down towards the right extended leg along with one exhalation. Try to go as far as you can in your comfort level. Put your hand on the right ankle or shin wherever you can reach. Left hand remains above the head. Hold it for a few seconds. Breathe normally (always remember never hold your breath in any exercise during pregnancy and never try to overstretch your body). Take your hands up into an upright position and repeat the same for left leg side (Fig. 4.7). This is a very good exercise for your middle and lower back pain as it makes the

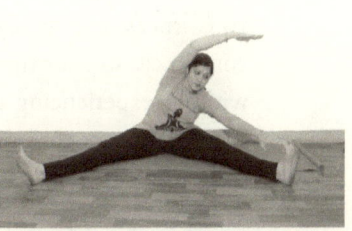

spine more strong and flexible. It also strengthens and firms the abdominal and legs muscles. It provides stimulating effect to the abdominal organs and improves digestion.

Back Stretch

- Sit in a Vajrasana on a mat, keeping your back straight. Take a deep breath and raise both your hands above your head. Then gradually bend forward to rest your forehead on the mat with hands outstretched. Hold the stretch for a few seconds and then come back. Repeat it for 5–6 times (Fig. 4.8).

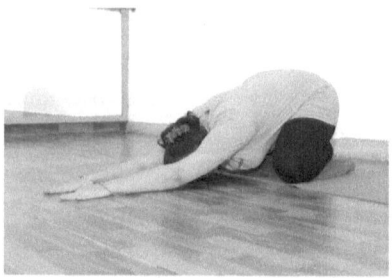

- As your pregnancy advances, you find this movement a little difficult. At that stage, you widen your knees and increase the space between both your knees so your tummy can adjust in that space without experiencing any pressure over abdomen. You can sit on a firm pillow or on a block to reduce strain on your knees and ankles.
- This exercise improves flexibility in legs and knees, releases tension in the shoulder and arms, and stretches and strengthens your spine and back muscles.

Floor Exercises in Lying Position (Back Exercises)

Bridging

- In pregnancy, you are supposed to do half or short bridge. Lie down on your back, preferably on a yoga mat. Bend your knees but keep a short distance between them. Feet flat on the floor and hands should be at sides. Now raise your lower back and hips off the floor so that there is a straight line between the shoulders and feet. Don't over-arch your back. While holding this pose, if it is comfortable to you, lift your toes so that the balls of feet are off the floor and you are working on your shin muscles to prevent cramp in the calf muscles. Flatten your feet and come out of the bridge position slowly (Fig. 4.9).

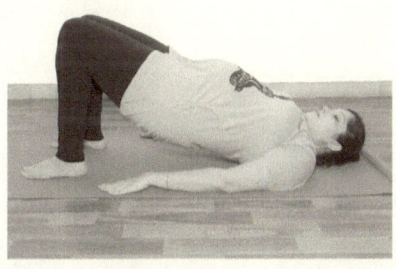

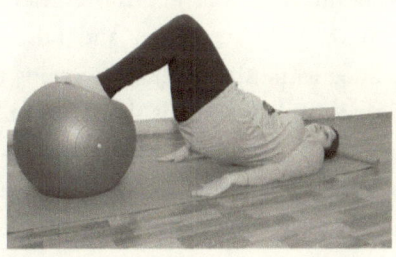

- Bridging exercise is sometimes useful to turn the breech babies (a breech baby lies in the uterus with feet facing the cervix); however, it does not work all the times.
- It strengthens the whole back muscles and thus eliminates or minimises your back pain.
- It also tones up and tightens the thighs.

Variation (On Exercise Ball)

Herein keep your legs straight. Put an exercise ball under your feet so your legs will be in slanting position.

Press your heels on the ball and lift your hips off, keeping the shoulders and head on the mat. Now bring your knees towards your chest by rolling the ball and keeping the hips lifted if possible. Finally, lower your hips, straighten your legs, and roll the ball back. This exercise helps in prevention of poor posture.

Arms and Legs Rising

- Lie on your back with both the knees folded and feet flat on the floor. Clasp your hands keeping the shoulders relaxed. Now with one deep inhalation, raise your hands overhead and stretch. Simultaneously straighten and raise one leg off the floor while the other leg remains in the same position. Both the thighs should be in line to each other.
- Hold there for a few seconds and feel stretch in your shoulders and upper back. Breathing should be normal.
- Bring down your hands, feet back on the floor, breathe out completely, and relax (Fig. 4.10).

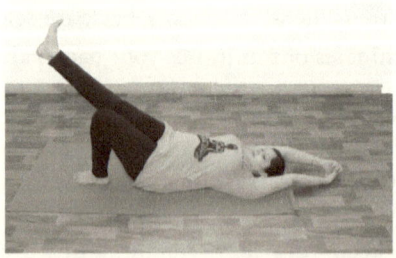

- Repeat the same with the other leg.

- In this exercise, you are working on your hands, legs, and back simultaneously. It strengthens your core muscles and improves your pelvic stability.
- Your abdominals also come in action here and thus get tone up.

Leg Curls

- Lie on your back, with both the knees completely bent and feet flat on the floor. Keep a fair distance between both the feet. Hand spread out away from the body. Take 2–3 abdominal breaths. Now rotate both the legs to one side (say, right), don't lift your feet off the floor and try to touch the floor with your knees. Turn your face to the left (opposite) side (Fig. 4.11).

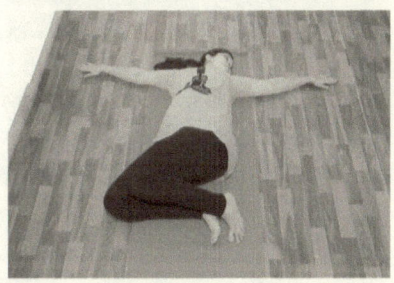

- Feel the stretch in the lower back and hips. Hold it for 5 seconds then repeat on the other side. This exercise can be done on the exercise ball also. This is a very good exercise for lower back pain. It gives massaging effect and release tension from the lower back. It helps to tone up the thigh, buttocks, and waist.

Leg Lifts in Side Lying

- Lie on the mat on your one side with your shoulder, hip, knee, and ankle in a straight line. Bend your bottom leg at 90° or at the angle that stabilise you on the mat and provide better balance. Keeping your top leg straight, lift it towards the ceiling. Keep breathing normally. Lower your leg slowly and repeat the up and down movement of leg 8–10 times (Fig. 4.12).

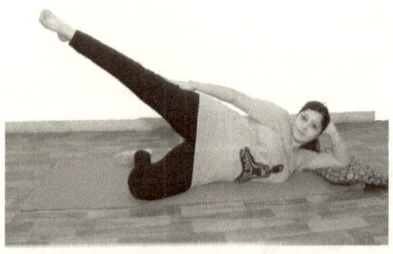

- In the same position, move your top leg from the hip joint side to side (pendulum movement). Remember to keep your knee straight and ensure that your hip remains parallel and in line with your shoulder throughout the motion. Repeat this side-to-side movement 8–10 times.
- Change the side and do both the exercises on the other leg.
- This exercise strengthens your hip muscles, tones up and tightens the thigh muscles, and helps relieving lower backache.

Spinal Rotation

- Lie down on your left side with a pillow or folded towel under your head. Slide both the knees up towards your tummy so that there should be 90° angle between your thigh and leg bone.
- Stretch both the arms and allow them to lie out in front of you. Remember to keep your shoulder blades down and lower back in neutral. Inhale and bring your right (top) hand up, follow your palm with your eyes so that your head will also turn in that direction comfortably.
- As you breathe out, open your right shoulder, taking your hand and arm away behind you completely so that your right palm touches the floor. Feel the stretch in your shoulder and upper back (Fig. 4.13).

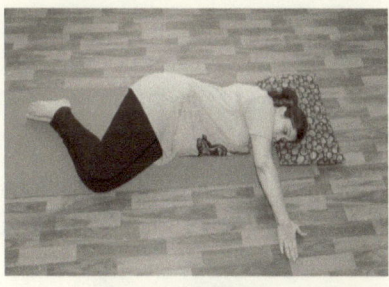

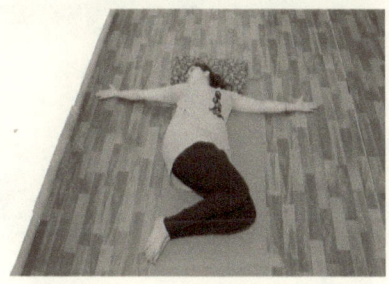

- Repeat this exercise on the other side too.

Floor Exercises in Kneeling Position

Cat and Camel Pose

- This exercise is done in all four positions on your hands and knees. Your wrist should be directly under your shoulders and knees are directly under your hips. Spread out your fingers and palms flat on the mat. Now working at your abdominal muscles, arch your spine upward towards the ceiling like a camel hump and your face should be down. Hold it for 3 seconds then slowly relax your back (Fig. 4.14, 4.15).

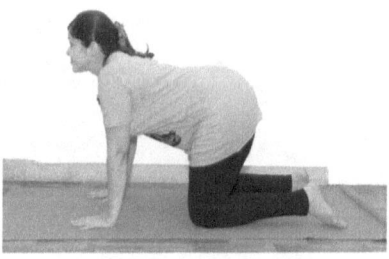

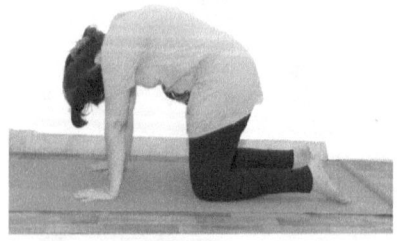

- Now allow your stomach fall towards the floor and make your back concave. As you do this, your head will lift up towards the ceiling.
- Continue doing both the poses very swiftly, no jerky movements should be done.
- You can incorporate breathing with this. Inhale when you look up (in cat pose) and exhale in camel pose.
- Cat and camel pose strengthens your lower abdominal muscles and reduces the stress from the lower spine. It also supports the uterus and very helpful exercise during labour.
- In the last month of pregnancy, if your baby has not turned in head down position, you can encourage the baby to rotate by adapting all four positions.

Variation

- This exercise can also be done in the sitting position.
- Sit on a firm mattress or yoga mat with the legs straight. Bend your knees and hold them with your hands. Now push your body backside making a hump (convex) in your back. Head should be down and hands completely outstretched from the elbow.
- Keep your hands on your knees. After holding there for a few seconds, come forward with your chest expanding and making a concave curve in your back. Shoulder should be retracted and head up. Keep hands on your knees and slightly bend from the elbow.
- Inhale when your head up and chest expanded. Exhale when your head down (in camel hump pose).

Arm and Leg Lift (Dynamic Diagonal Stretch)

- Same starting position as in cat and camel pose (all four pose). Simultaneously lift your right arm in front of you and left leg back side in completely stretched posture. If you are not able to do it, first lift right arm balance your body and then lift left leg. Hold this superwoman pose for 5 seconds, and then repeat with left arm and right leg. Keep your elbow and knee straight. Try to lift both to the same height as you are making a line (Fig. 4.16).

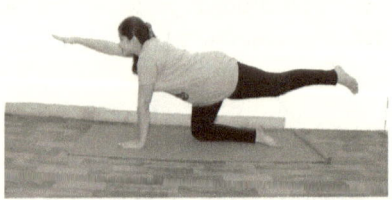

- In between the two moves, just rotate you buttocks in circular motion (clockwise then anti-clockwise) to release tension from the lower back and feel relaxation.
- This exercise works on and strengthens the core muscles and improves core stability. It helps in correcting the poor posture. In diagonal stretch, balancing on one hand and knee provides the base for full body extension and will help you to develop the sense of balance. It maintains good working relationship between the upper and lower body. You wonder that this kind of stretch creates more growing space for the baby.

Resting Pose

- After the above two sequences (cat and camel and diagonal stretch), just rest your body down in an extended cat pose. Sit on your knees and heels, bend forward, and put your head down on the floor. Herein you have to keep a fair distance between both the knees so that your tummy can adjust in between that width.
- Head is down and forehead is touching the floor. Rest your arms on the floor in front of you, elbows slightly bent so that there is no tension or stretch in the hands. Hold this pose for a few breaths.
- This is a very relaxing pose for pregnant women, especially for those who have the urge to lie on their tummy. (Refer fig. 4.8.)

Standing Moves (For Stretching and Flexibility)

Chest Expansion with Shoulder Stretch

- Stand erect with feet apart (at least 2–3 feet distance between them). Keep your feet parallel to each other, toes facing forward, not outward. Your legs should be firmly gripped to the ground.
- Tuck you tummy in and straighten yourself as you are getting taller. Clasp your hands behind you. Stretch your hands up behind, taking them away from the body. Simultaneously bend your body forward from the hips. Go down so that your back becomes parallel to the floor. Raise your head up and look forward. Remember to

keep your knees and elbows straight and keep breathing normally.

- Hold this pose for a few seconds or depending on your comfort level. Then slowly come back into the standing position.

- Once you get grip on this exercise, you can combine the forward-bending movement with the side-stretching movements.

- This exercise releases the stiffness and tension from the neck, shoulder, and back. Just do this stretching exercise when you feel tired or upset as its positive effects may help you to lift your mood and energise you. It opens up the lungs and chest area and thus improves your respiration. It also lifts your breasts and prevents them from sagging.

Arms Stretching (Warrior Pose)

- In yoga, it is called 'Virbhadrasana'. Stand with feet wide apart (minimum 3 feet distance), press down your heels to the ground firmly. Your feet should face forward and parallel to each other. Now turn your right foot out completely (at 90°) and turn left foot slightly inside.

- Open your arms out and raise them slightly above the shoulder level. Palms are facing down.

- Now, to move into an 'archer pose', bend your right knee up to the point where your knee and ankle come in a straight vertical line. Look at your right hand.

- Remember to keep both the hands and your left leg completely extended. Distribute your body weight equally on both feet (Fig. 4.17). Hold the pose for 3 breaths. Come into your starting position. Put your hands down if they are fatigued. Repeat the same on the left side.

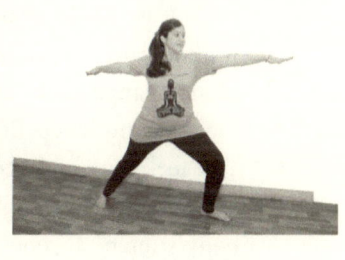

- This yoga pose opens up your chest and lungs, thus increases your breathing capacity. It strengthens you physically and mentally and builds up your stamina and concentration. It develops your balance and stability. It stretches and strengthens your whole lower extremities.

Whole Body Stretch

- Stand directly in front of a wall or a fixed rod if you have. Place your hands on the wall or hold the rod. Hands should be in line with your shoulder.
- Walk behind away from the wall and simultaneously bend from the hip joint; 90° angle should be formed at hip joint. Your neck and back should be parallel to the floor. Don't bend your elbow at any point (Fig. 4.18).

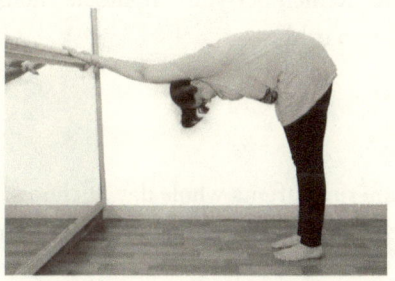

- You feel a fantastic stretch in your shoulder, arms, thighs, back, and in calf muscles. Hold the pose for at least 12–15 seconds to get the benefit. Slowly walk towards the wall, raise your head and body up. Don't change your position in a hurry.
- Do a few more repetitions.
- You feel your body completely free from stiffness and relaxed after completing a few sets of 'whole body stretch'. It tones up your arms, back, thighs, and calf muscles.

Pelvic Rotation (Belly Dancing)

- This is a favourite movement for most of the pregnant women.
- Stand up straight with feet slightly apart. Place your hands below your waist. Preferably do this exercise in front of a mirror. Rotate your pelvic in a circular move as you are making circles with your hips. Incorporate the forward and backwards pelvic tilt along with.
- Do this rhythmic circular movement in one direction (clockwise) making around 20 circles. Then another 20 circles in the opposite direction (anti-clockwise). Keep your breathing at normal pace. Remember your shoulders should not move with your hips.

Benefits

If you are tired after a whole day of chores, this exercise helps in relieving tired, aching muscles. It increases the mobility in your lower back, hips, and pelvis. It alleviates your low back pain and discomforts of pregnancy.

PARTNER/COUPLE YOGA

According to studies, pregnancy is the 12th most stressful events of the life. The stress causing factors are changed body image, hormonal mood swings, decreased sexual interest, stress about future mothering responsibilities, decreased self-esteem if you have stopped working, etc.

Here, partner can play a very important role in developing the self-awareness and faith in her. Fatherhood role doesn't start only after the birth of baby, but he can actively participate in her antenatal program too. This involvement increases the love and bonding not only between the couple, but also with your unborn baby.

Couple yoga is a unique healing art, the realm of relationship and authentic connection with your partner. Here, you both can simply assist each other in which essentially you do adjustments on each other. Unlike practicing alone, couple work is deeply rooted on a shared experience. You can also practice partner yoga with your friend, sister, or other colleague at your antenatal class.

1. **Double-sided stretch pose:** Stand on either side of your partner at a distance of about 3 feet. Bring your both feet together and stand tall. Bend towards your partner and bring your partner sided hand to rest on the other's hip, while the opposite hands of both the partner should be overhead and hold each

other at wrist or elbow level. Apply little force into their hip as if you are trying to push them away and simultaneously pulling overhead hand in your direction. Thus you can feel a deep, opening side stretch. Then interchange your positions and do it for the other side.

2. **Twin tree pose:** Begin by standing a few feet apart with your partner, facing the same direction. Bring your opposite palms together into a 'Namaste mudra'. Shift the weight onto your right feet and draw the left leg into a tree pose by bending the knee and bringing the left foot to the inner thigh of standing (right) leg. Your partner will shift weight onto left foot and bring the right foot to the inner thigh of left leg. Lift your partner sided hand overhead and hold each other there (Fig. 4.19). Help to balance each other for at least 4–5 breaths and then release. Turn around or change your standing direction to repeat on other side.

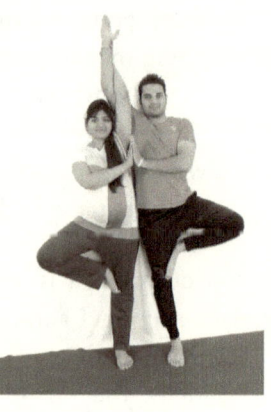

3. **Diagonal stretch in kneeling:** Same position as we earlier discussed in 'cat and camel pose', but here both the partners are facing each other. Keep one hand distance between you. Both of you will lift your right hand and left leg simultaneously. Stretch right hand as much forward and rest it onto your partner's left shoulder. Keep your head up and look

into each other's eyes. Feel the love, support, and safety for each other. Hold it for 2–3 breaths and repeat it on opposite side.

4. **Forward stretch:** Sit opposite or facing each other with your legs extended in a broad V shape. Bring the soles of your feet in contact with your partner's feet. Extend your arms towards each other and hold it at the wrist level. Bend forward from the hips towards your partner, keeping your spine and arms straight. At the same time, your partner pulls his body backwards. Feel stretch in your legs and back. Hold there for a few seconds. Then your partner will bend forward and you extend your back. Do a few repetitions. This is a good hamstrings (thigh muscles) stretching exercise (Fig. 4.20).

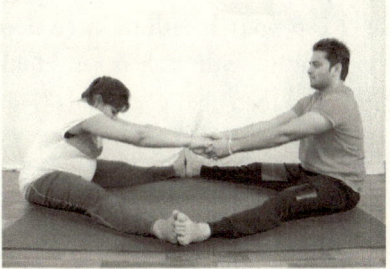

5. **Dancing duo:** Stand facing each other. Hold each other's right hands. Both of you soften through knees and shift weight onto right leg. Bend left knee and hold your left foot or ankle with your left hand. Gently press left leg onto your left hand and feel stretch in front of your left thigh. Both partners should hold each other's right hand in front to balance in a dancer's pose. Gaze at each other

and enjoy this stretchful moment. Hold it and then repeat on the other side.

6. **Partner twist:** This is called 'Ardhamatsyendrasana'. This seated twist is very easy, but an intimate movement when performed with partner. Sit back to back and cross-legged. Your spine is completely in contact with partner's spine. Inhale and take your arms up over the head holding each other's hand or wrists and start to lengthen the spine. Exhale and twist to the right. Bring your right hand to the inside of your partner's left knee and your left hand to the outside of your right knee. This applies to both the partners, so the pose is like a mirror image. With every inhalation, lengthen your spine and find more space, and with each exhalation, try to twist your body a bit more utilising your partner's knee. Keep your breathing pace normal and try to synchronise with each other. Hold it for a few seconds and then change the side (Fig. 4.21).

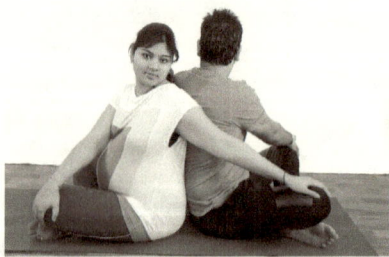

7. **Partner breathing:** After doing all these stretching poses, now time to relax and connect with each other. Start in a seated position with leg crossed and with your back resting against each other (be a human wall for each other). You can either sit in a 'vajrasana' or in

a half 'padmasana' if it is comfortable and relaxing for both of you. Rest your hands on the thighs. Allow yourself to completely indulge in this moment and feel a strong bond with your partner (Fig. 4.22). Close your eyes and begin to 'breathe alternate' with your partner. As you inhale, he exhales; and as he inhales, you exhale. Continue breathing and remain in the pose for at least 10 minutes. This is a very spiritual pose which opens up your heart and feel the closeness to your partner as if you are one unit.

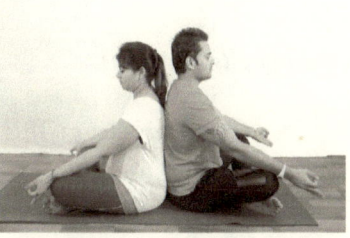

STRENGTHENING EXERCISES

Dumbbells and TheraBand Exercises

Many women don't realize the importance of upper-body strength during pregnancy. Actually your shoulders, arms, upper back will be used extensively during the first year of childbirth. You need strong arm and shoulder muscles to carry your growing baby for long hours.

Upper-body strengthening exercises tone up and firm your arms. It strengthens your shoulders, neck, chest, and upper back. It also improves and maintains good body posture. Dumbbell exercises are to be done in standing posture, but if you are not comfortable, then sit on a straight backed sturdy chair. Do 8–10 repetition for all the exercises.

Remember, the dumbbells and band exercises should be done only twice or thrice in a week. Start with 500 g or 1 kg weight in both the hands, whichever is comfortable for you. Do not exceed more than 1.5 kg.

Dumbbells Exercises

- **Shoulder shrug:** This is just a shoulder-shrugging exercise to start with. Stand erect with your feet slightly apart. Hold dumbbells in both hands. Shoulders should be pushed downward and relaxed. Now raise both your shoulders up towards your ears and then release. Don't do jerky movements. Inhale while you raise and exhale while dropping down.

- **Biceps raises:** Stand erect and maintain your body alignment or sit straight on a chair. Hold dumbbells and turn your elbows so that your palms facing the front side. Inhale and bring the weights up to your shoulders. Then exhale and take your weights above the head. Without holding there more, inhale again and bring the weights down to the shoulders and lastly take them back to the starting position with a long relaxing exhalation with mouth. Remember, to maintain your back arch and continue it again with a rhythm (Fig. 4.23).

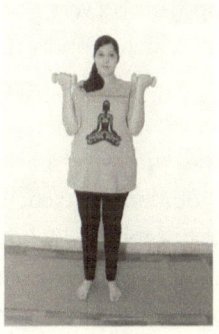 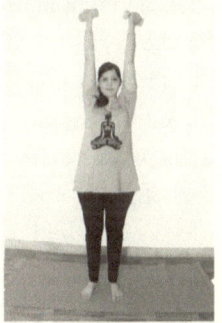

- **Chest opener**: Stand with your proper body alignment. Hold the dumbbells or weights. Your hands should be at the sides. Take one deep breath and extend your hands in front of you at the shoulder level. Check both the hands are parallel and just breathe out. From that position, inhale and draw both the arms opposite to each other (take them towards the sides) so that you feel that your shoulder blades (scapulas) are coming towards each other. Do not sway back and don't bend your

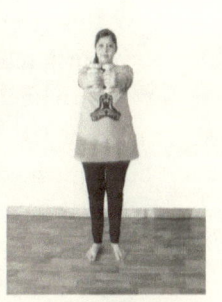

elbows when you are extending the arms at sides. Exhale and take them in front of you again (Fig. 4.24). Inhale and take the hands away, exhale and bring them together in front of you. Remember to keep your shoulders

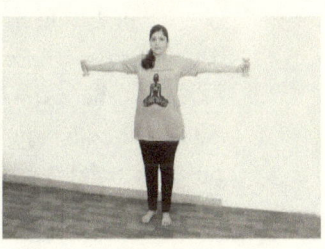

relaxed, not hunched up. This is a very good exercise for the pectoral muscles which support the breasts. Thus it tones up and firms the breasts and prevents them from sagging.

- **Triceps exercise:** Stand with your back straight, feet slightly apart, shoulders relaxed, and chin tucked in. Hold 1 kg dumbbells in both hands. Extend your arms straight up above your head. Upper arms should touch the earlobes. Inhale and bend your elbows back side so that dumbbells will touch the cervical region. Exhale and straighten the elbows, but don't bring your shoulder down. Repeat for at least 8 times. Then slowly bring both the hands down. After this exercise, just swing your hands back and forth with weights in your hands. This gives the traction pull in your shoulder joint which relieves any kind of stiffness or adhesion.

- **Dumbbell floor press:** Lie on your back with knees bent and feet flat on the floor. Hold the dumbbell in each hand. Bend your elbows in and keep a 90° angle between your upper arm and forearm. Elbows should be rested on the floor. Now push your hands straight up, bringing the dumbbells directly over your chest. Then bring them back to the sides. Again inhale and push the weights up; exhale and return back (Fig. 4.25).

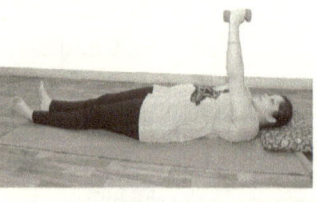

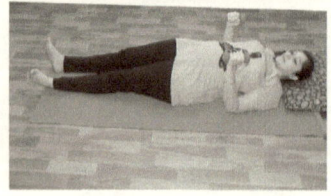

This exercise builds up your chest muscles and shoulder blade muscles.

■ **Twist and punch:** Stand erect in proper alignment. Hold 1 kg dumbbells in both the hands, legs slightly apart. Bend your elbows and retract the shoulders back so that you can hold the dumbbells at your waist level. Now turn your upper body to the left while pushing the right leg away and straighten your right elbow as if you are punching someone to your left with dumbbell. Inhale and come back. Do it same on the opposite side. Turn upper body to the right, and punch with your left arm. Inhale and return to starting position. Remember to keep your back and knee straight and other shoulder retracted (Fig. 4.26).

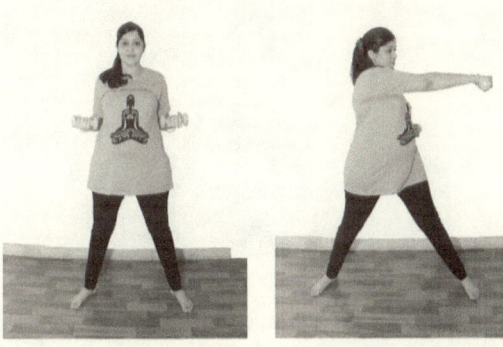

Resistance Band Exercises

For strengthening exercises with TheraBand or resistance band, initially choose low-resistance band. Don't do all the dumbbells and band exercises in a single day, choose either of them.

- **Reverse fly:** Either you can stand or just sit on an exercise ball. For more stability, you can sit on an armless chair. Cross the resistance band passing under your feet. Feet should be shoulder-width apart. Keep your spine and head in neutral comfortable position (or you can slightly bend forward from your chest). Palms of the hands are facing each other and keep your elbow slightly bent. Take a breath in and open both the arms from the shoulder, take them away from the body. Exhale and take your hands back near the body in a slow, controlled manner. Repeat the same for 8–10 times. This exercise strengthens your shoulder blade muscles and also tones up your breasts (Fig. 4.27).

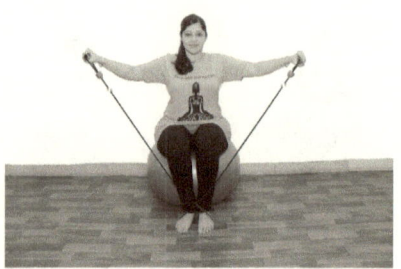

- **Slide and squat:** Stand with your legs together, but knees and toes slightly turned outward. Hold the resistance band with both hands overhead. Hold the band from the centre, but keep some distance between both hands. Now take your right foot away to the right side and immediately

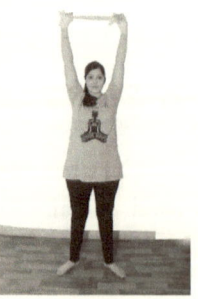

come in a half squat position. Simultaneously stretch the band in your hand wide and pull it down towards your back. Exhale and bring your right foot back and take the band overhead again in the starting position (Fig. 4.28). Do five repetitions 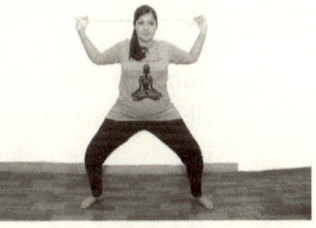 with right leg and five to the left leg. Squats will strengthen your inner thighs and hips. With the resistance band, you will make your arms strong.

- **Side walk:** In a standing position, keep your legs together and parallel to each other. Cross the band from your front passing under your feet and hold it with both your hands. Band should be of equal length from both sides. Maintain your shoulders slightly retracted and chest lifted. Now step your right leg out to the right side, followed by the left leg as if you are walking sideways. Then take out the left leg to the left side followed by the right leg. Keep walking sideways with the resistance, thus you strengthen your inner and outer thigh muscles and buttocks (Fig. 4.29).

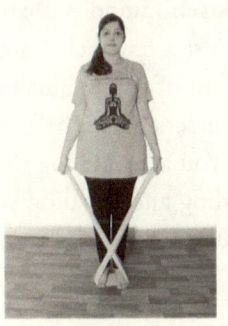
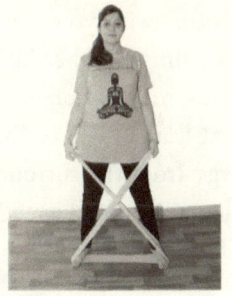

- **Bicep curls:** Secure your TheraBand underneath your feet and with your hands in front of the thighs. Keep your arms straight and palms facing up. Now pull the band towards your shoulder by bending from the elbow and then slowly straighten the elbow in the starting position. Remember to keep your back erect, shoulders relaxed, and upper arms immobile throughout the movement.

SALUTE TO BABY

Sun salutation or Surya Namaskar is a compiled set of 12 yoga postures that provide a good cardiovascular workout. It is an important fundamental flowing yoga sequence that energises your body as you stretch and strengthen all of the major muscle groups.

Just like Sun salutation, Baby salute is a long-established skilled concept in the prenatal fitness. It is a combination of some of the important yoga asana. If you do not have much time and energy, you can practice this short sequence daily and thus prepare yourself both physically and mentally for the amazing birth experience.

Position I (starting pose): Stand up straight in Tadasana with your feet just a few inches apart. Place your palms together in front of you (Namaste mudra). In the same position now, practice some belly breathing. Do at least 6–8 breaths. You are inhaling the positive energy from the surrounding and exhaling your stress and anxiety out (Fig. 4.30).

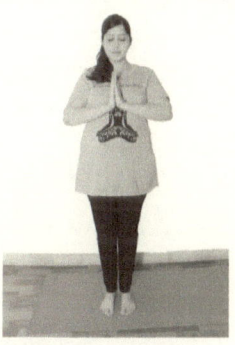

II (spinal rotation): From the Namaskar mudra, now stretch both your hands out in front of you, keeping your palms together. Widen your legs. Then with a deep inhalation, take your right arm behind you, keeping the elbow straight. Turn your face and body towards the right side along with the right hand. Hold it there and do 2–3 pant blow out through your mouth. Come back and bring your right hand in front of you. Again inhale and take your left arm behind. Repeat the same to your left side. You will feel stretching across your shoulders. You can repeat this move for a couple of times. Release your arms and bring them down to move to the next stretch.

III (cradle): Inhale and bring your arms in front of you at the shoulder level taking hold of each to opposite elbow—cradle position (right hand on the left elbow and left hand on right elbow). Exhale and bend forward from the hips (back should be straight), spreading your legs slightly apart and outward rotated. Keeping your back straight and legs strong, inhale and turn to your right side as far as you can. Exhale and come back to the centre. Inhale and turn left, exhale and back to centre. Repeat this side-to-side movement gracefully as you are holding and rocking your baby in your arms. After a few repetitions, release your arms and stand straight (Fig 4.31).

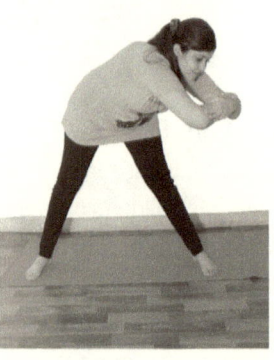

IV (squatting): Keeping your legs in same position (wide apart), raise your hands in front of you with palms facing down. Exhale and bend your knees to come in to a complete squat sitting position. Your feet flat on the floor, and join hands in Anjali (Namaste) mudra near your chest. Your right elbow should be supported on the right knee and left elbow on the left knee. Remember to extend your spine long and breathe normally. If possible, do abdominal breathing in this pose. Inhale and feel that the air is going directly to your baby through your navel. You can exhale through your mouth (pursed lip breathing) to relieve your stress and get relaxed (Fig. 4.32).

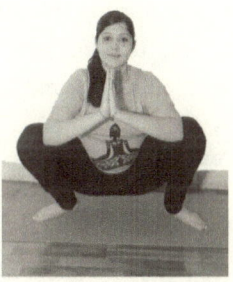

In the last months of pregnancy, if you find it difficult to do abdominal breathing in squatting position, just widen your legs little more and focus on the pelvic floor tightening (Kegel exercise). Make your pelvic floor muscles tight, hold, and relax. Do a few repetitions but never hold your breathing in between.

V (butterfly movement): Now with the support of your hands, slowly put your buttocks down and sit in a butterfly position. The soles of the feet should touch each other and hold your ankles with your hands. Move your knees up and down in a slow, rhythmic manner. This will stretch your inner thigh muscles. At last, rest your knees on the mat if possible (Buddha konansana). In the same position, lower your head down towards your feet as much as you can. Inhale and come up slowly. Again exhale and bend forward. Do it for a few breaths. (Refer fig. 4.4)

VI (sitting side stretch): From the butterfly position, now slowly turn your right knee inward so that it touches the left foot sole. This is Z sitting position. Place both your hands on the mat on your sides. Inhale and bring your right arm over the head. As you breathe out, lengthen your right side and bend towards your left side as far as you feel comfortable and get a little stretch. Then release and take the arm down. Now change your leg positions and repeat the same on the other side.

VII (cat and camel): Put both your hands on the mat in front of you and slowly come into all fours or crawling position. Your shoulders should be exactly above your wrists, and hips should be above your knees. Do some cat and camel tilts swiftly to relieve your back strain. (Refer fig. 4.15.)

VIII (leg stretch and knee bend): In crawling position, slightly shift your body weight on left leg and straighten your right leg out behind you. Place the right foot down on the mat, and try to lower the heel as much as you can. Feel the nice stretch in your calf. Now take your right foot off the floor, straighten your right leg up in the air, and then bend from the knee at around 90° angle. Keep your back straight and feel the stretch into the groin region. Then slowly put your leg and knee down to the mat in the starting position (all fours). Repeat this leg stretch and knee bend movement on the left leg. If you are comfortable, repeat this for a few more times. Remember to breathe normally and never overexert or overstretch your body (Fig. 4.33).

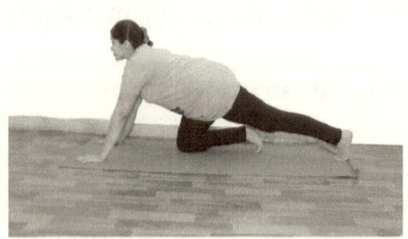

IX (relaxation pose): In crawling position, widen up your knees (increase the space between your knees) and bring your feet together as you are making letter V with your legs. Push your body forward and let your hands bear your upper-body weight. Keep your elbows straight and fingers widely spread on the mat. Do not drop or arch your back and keep your head in neutral position. Your weight should be transferred to both hands equally. Now slowly release the pressure from your hands, come backwards, sit on your heels, and extend your arms straight over your head. Rest your head down on the floor. As you have widened your knees, your expanded tummy will be accommodated in the space between your knees. Stay in the pose for a few breaths. Your back pressure will be relieved and you feel completely relaxed in this position. (Refer fig. 4.8.)

X (vajrasana): Slowly raise your head and body up from the previous relaxation pose and sit straight on the heels in a Vajrasana pose. If you are uncomfortable, use pillow under your knees and between your thighs and legs. Do some abdominal or baby breathing in this pose. Now interlock your fingers. Inhale and stand on your knees, simultaneously take both arms up over your head. Try to stretch your hands more and feel the length in your spine. Breathe out, take your hands down, and sit on your heels again (in Vajrasana). Repeat it for 5–6 times. (Refer fig. 4.6.)

XI (lunge position): Keep a pillow below your knees so your knees don't get hurt. From a Vajrasana position, lift your buttocks and stand on your knees (kneeling pose). Now lift your left knee and extend the left lower leg forward. Place the sole of left foot on the mat. Your thigh and shin should be perpendicular to each other. Your hands should be either on the lower waist or on your left thigh. Now, gradually bend your left knee little forward and shift your body weight to the left leg. Your back should be straight and tailbone tucked. If you can keep your balance, now lift the right foot off the floor as you make V with your right thigh and right shin. Hold for a few seconds and release. Change your leg positions and repeat it on the other leg. This pose looks like a 'peacock pose'.

XII (kneel to stand): From the kneeling position, your next move is the standing pose. Place both your hands on your front thighs. Keep your head and back neutral. With your hand support, slowly get up in a standing posture (Tadasana). Join your palms in front of your chest and breathe normally.

XIII (ending pose): Raise your hands up over your head with palms joining each other (Namaste mudra). Look upward to your hands and stretch the hands little more from the shoulders as you are getting taller. Then separate your hands to sides, take them away from each other, turn your palms down, and bring the hands back to the side. Repeat a couple of times. Inhale and raise your hands up, exhale, and bring them down (Fig 4.34).

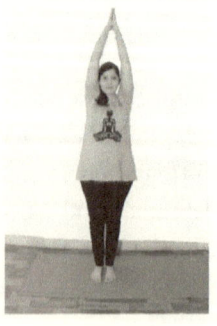

End up the series with a nice thought of your baby, as this is the 'salute to baby'. With practice, you will develop flexibility, strength, and endurance in your body. Initially it is advisable to learn and practice this under the guidance of your antenatal therapist.

5

Nutritional Baggage

It is a dream of every mother to give birth to a healthy baby. To fulfil your dream, first you need to understand the importance of different food groups. You should understand and follow the healthy diet with its right quantity which satisfies the nutritional requirements of the baby as well as your own body. Armed with the proper exercise program, medical assistance, and a perfect diet planning, your road to the destination will surely be as smooth as it can be.

A healthy diet is an important part of everyone's life, but it is especially vital during pregnancy. You should know the proper nutritional values of the food you are taking because your eating habits directly affect your baby. A balanced diet plan during pregnancy will give your baby a strong start in its life. Nutritional evaluation is very important before and during pregnancy as well as after birth too (for an effective breastfeeding). An inadequate amount of some nutrients may cause malformation, medical problems, low birth weight, or some neurological disorders in the foetus. Nutritional deficit or haphazard diet intake affects mother's body too and she may suffer from digestive disturbances, anaemia, fatigue, cramps, gestational diabetes, or preeclampsia. A well-nourished body can bounce back faster and more easily after delivery. Even though you are taking prenatal vitamins, it is essential that you get enough vitamins and other nutrients from the food you eat. So your goal is to ensure that you are eating food with each of the necessary nutrients from each of the food groups every day.

Most pregnant mothers need only 300–400 extra calories per day in their diet, which is equivalent of 480 ml of low-fat milk or 250 gm of ice cream. Doctors recommend 3 healthy meals a day—breakfast, lunch, and dinner—and 3 smaller snacks in between. So you need to eat a total of 6 times a day. Frequent smaller meals help in controlling your blood sugar level which is important for healthy mom and developing baby. According to the American College of Obstetrics and Gynaecologist (ACOG), the pregnant woman should eat the following amounts daily (Fig.5.1):

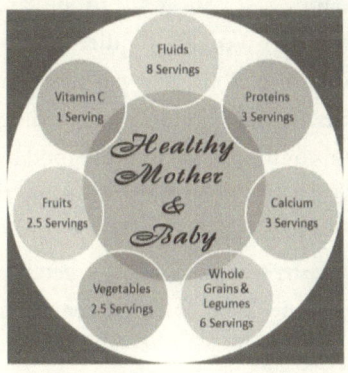

- 6–7 servings of rice or whole bread/pasta (carbohydrates)
- 3 servings of vegetables (vitamins)
- 3 servings of fruits (vitamins and minerals)
- 3–4 servings of dairy milk, yoghurt, paneer/cheese (calcium)
- 3 servings of pulses, nuts, beans (protein) (1 serving = ½ cup)

What Are the Essential Nutrients

- **Folic acid:** Folic acid is actually vitamin B9 which is most beneficial during the first month after conception when the neural tube development starts. But unfortunately many women don't realize they are pregnant during their first month. So folic acid supplement should begin prior to the conception and continue throughout the pregnancy. Folic acid helps in the development of foetal brain and spine. It prevents birth defects like cleft lip and palate, neural tube defect, and spina bifida.

  Folic acid enhances the production of RBC (red blood cells) in your body. This is vital during pregnancy as you tend to be anaemic during this phase. Women require approximately 600 microgram of folic acid per day throughout the 9 months. It may be hard to get the recommended amount of folic acid from the food alone. You need to take some supplements according to your doctor's prescription.

  Food sources: green leafy vegetables like spinach and kale, fortified cereals and bread, and lentils, corn, carrot, beans, papaya, peas, bottle gourd, grape fruits, oranges

- **Calcium:** You will need enough calcium to strengthen your bones and teeth as well as to build up strong bones and teeth in your baby. Calcium helps your baby to grow a healthy heart, nerves, and muscles and also helps to develop blood-clotting abilities.

  Pregnant women of the age of 19 and above need 1,000 mg of calcium per day, an increase of 400 mg a day over your usual needs. Calcium with multivitamin supplements is to be taken when milk products are less in your daily diet. Calcium supplements work best with the vitamin D (best source of vitamin D is early morning sunlight). Vitamin D increases the absorption of calcium.

  ***Food sources*:** milk, yoghurt, cottage cheese, tofu broccoli, banana, spinach, roasted almonds and sesame seeds, soya and fruit juices/smoothie/pudding

- **Iron:** Iron is a crucial component which provides more oxygen to our organs and tissues. In pregnancy, you need extra iron for the formation of haemoglobin in the blood, which ultimately supplies oxygen to your baby. Many Indian women are suffering from anaemia nowadays, so plenty of iron during pregnancy is a must for you and your baby.

  Lack of iron may lead to fatigue and depression in mother, preterm delivery, and low birth weight of baby. The daily recommended dose of iron is 25–30 mg.

Food sources: green leafy vegetables like spinach,
fenugreek, broccoli, fish, red meat, fortified
cereals, dried fruits like raisins, fig, and apricots,
apples, beetroot, mushroom and legumes

As your pregnancy progresses, your doctor will prescribe you the iron tablets, as the requirements increase in the later months. In many pregnant mothers, iron does not get absorbed easily, so they are advised to consume it with vitamin C rich food as vitamin C is known to increase the absorption of iron by up to 6 times. So it is recommended to take the iron tablet with orange or strawberry juice in the morning as they are absorbed better on an empty stomach. Consume more fibre-rich foods when you are on iron supplements, because iron has a tendency to upset your GI tract and harden the stool and thus lead to constipation.

- **Protein:** Protein is very important for the development of uterus and breasts in the mother. Protein is made up of amino acid which is the building block of your body's cells formation and of your baby's body as well. It plays a major role in your baby's development as it grows from a single-cell to a multi-celled organism. Protein is also essential in the production of some hormones and enzymes. Pregnant women require plenty of protein (at least 75 gm) daily and especially during 2nd and 3rd trimester.

Food sources: eggs, lean meat, fish, lentils, beans,
sprouts, pulses, nuts especially peanuts,
tofu, soy

- **Carbohydrates:** They are the main energy source for the immediate use in day-to-day metabolism. Carbohydrates include simple sugars like glucose, galactose, and fructose; disaccharides like sucrose, maltose, and lactose; and complex plant starch like whole grain, oatmeal, sweet potatoes, bananas, apricots, and peach.

  Avoid processed and refined foods like white bread, white rice, soda, chips, cakes, and candy which contain more of simple carbohydrates. A simple carbohydrate is broken down quickly and leads to increase blood glucose and insulin level. These kind of high GI foods are responsible for the gestational diabetes.

  Low GI foods are the complex starches that are broken down slowly and keep your blood sugar level more stable. Some of the options are whole wheat, raagi (finger millet), jowar (sorghum), bajra (pearl/white millet), oats, sweet potatoes, etc.

- **Potassium:** Potassium is a mineral and electrolyte which supports muscles, nerves, and the electrical activities in the body. Excessive and prolonged vomiting may cause potassium deficiency. You might suffer from giddiness, muscles cramps, weakness, and constipation due to potassium deficiency.

  Food sources: fresh fruits, coconut water, potatoes meat, milk

- **Zinc:** It is a micronutrient and its deficiency may result in loss of appetite and low immunity. Zinc deficit may lead to IUGR (intra uterine growth retardation).

  Food sources: milk, low-fat yoghurt, cheddar cheese almonds, cashews, and peanuts, meat

- **Vitamin B complex:** The eight B vitamins (known as B complex) play an important role in supporting a healthy pregnancy. They keep your body strong while baby is growing inside your womb. Most important of all is vitamin B9 folic acid.

  Vitamin B complex deficiency leads to irritability, mouth ulcers, and tingling-numbness of the hands and feet. All the B complex vitamins are water soluble, so your body cannot store them. You need to consume it each and every day in order to get its benefit.

  Food sources: pulses, fish, eggs, meat, unprocessed whole grains and cereals, potatoes, bananas, chilli peppers

- **Vitamin C:** Vitamin C helps your body to absorb iron from the food, prevents your gum problems, constipation, and varicose vein. Pregnant mothers need 70–80 mg of vitamin C daily. Choose at least one good source of vitamin C every day such as all citrus fruits—oranges, strawberries, tomatoes, apricots, apples, grape fruits, and parsley.

- **Vitamin A:** Choose at least one source of vitamin A every alternate day. It is a fat-soluble vitamin and is stored in the liver and fat tissue. Vitamin A is good for the healthy skin and eyes, foetal growth, and immune system development. Vitamin A is very essential in the 3rd trimester as it promotes baby's lungs development and also helps mother with the postpartum repairs and recovery.

  Food sources: carrots, pumpkins, red and yellow peppers, mangoes, sweet potatoes, apricots, and tomatoes, eggs and fish

- **Vitamin D:** It promotes bone strength, immune functions, and healthy cell division. It is essential for the absorption and metabolism of calcium and phosphorus which help in the development of bones and teeth in the growing baby. You need 600 IU of vitamin D every day.

  Sources: main source of vitamin D is the sunlight fish, eggs, soy milk, orange juice, fortified cereals, tofu, mushrooms

- **Omega-3 fatty acid:** It is a powerful brain booster. Research has confirmed that adding omega-3 fatty acid to the diet of pregnant mothers have the positive effects on the visual and cognitive development of the baby. It reduces the risk of allergies in the infant, prevent preterm labour, and lower the risk of preeclampsia and depression in the mothers. Omega-3 fatty acids are also beneficial after the birth to make the breast milk.

  Food sources: fish oil, flex seeds, soy milk, eggs and dairy products, nuts especially walnut, finger millet (ragi)

- **Antioxidants:** Some of the micronutrients and vitamins are known to serve as antioxidants such as copper, zinc, manganese, vitamin A, vitamin C, and vitamin E. Antioxidants are the molecules which prevent or stop cell damage caused by the harmful oxidants (i.e., free radicals).

  Food sources: blueberries, papaya, spinach, red beans, tomatoes

It is advisable to take all the nutrients or supplements in required quantity. Do not go overboard. Sometimes higher level of some nutrients may cause digestive problems, kidney problems, and could hamper the absorption of other nutrients from the food into the blood.

Carbonated drinks make you dehydrated. Water is the best hydrating source in pregnancy. Water aids digestion, helps you to feel fresh, and maintains the amniotic fluid level in the amniotic sac. You should have minimum 10–12 glasses of water daily and this should be increased if you exercise or if you have a hectic day.

The placenta has amazing filtering properties, which shield your baby from the harmful nasty you may ingest. But research discovered that some pesticides slip through placenta and can be passed on to your baby. In fact, some amount of pesticide has been found in amniotic fluid, umbilical cord blood, and breast milk. So avoid eating outside at restaurants and hotels and prefer to eat fresh homemade food.

Six to eight ounce (200 ml) cup of tea, coffee, or soda per day won't be harmful, but it is advisable to avoid caffeine altogether if possible.

High consumption of caffeinated drinks leads to increase risk of miscarriage and other problems. So cut down your intake or switch to decaffeinated products. Raw eggs and raw fishes which are high in mercury like shark, swordfish should not be consumed. Unpasteurized milk, cheese, or juices should be avoided.

Weight Gain During Pregnancy

Ideal weight gain during pregnancy is 10–13 kg, but it varies in every pregnant woman. Your weight gain depends on a variety of factors such as your metabolism, your activity level, and your genetics. Some women start gaining their weight in the 1st trimester, or some may lose it because of hormonal changes and morning sickness. Don't worry, once your body adjusts with the hormones, your weight gain will pick up. Most of the mothers gain 1–2 kg weight during 1st trimester. Then during 2nd and 3rd trimester, steady gain is important for baby's proper growth and development, which should be about 1–2 kg per month. You should record your weight gain chart which helps you to manage your weight healthily.

If you are overweight, there are more chances of complications during pregnancy like high BP, gestational diabetes, or caesarean delivery. But this doesn't mean that you should go on fad diet or crash diet, because it will definitely harmful to you and your baby's growth. Instead of that, go for low calorie foods—avoid sugar, ice creams, chocolates, white breads, ghee, and butter. Increase the quantities of salads and fruits in your meal. Include some physical activities in your routine such as walk about 30 minutes every day, do exercise and yoga, and use stairs instead of the elevator.

If you are underweight and not gaining enough, it is also a cause of worry. Underweight women are at higher risk of preterm delivery or low birth weight. In such case, you need to increase your calorie intake. Take small meals/snacks frequently. Eat foods which are rich in good fats like peanut butter, olive oil, and nuts.

If you are suffering from nausea and vomiting and not able to eat adequate, then you should start to eat low carbohydrate diet. Drink lots of fluids in form of coconut water, buttermilk, curd, and non-citrus fruit shakes. Sometimes even the smells of certain foods cause the aversion. In cases, where your diet becomes too limited because of the aversion, try to find out some healthy food substitute to take their place. Take other medical supplements as prescribed by your doctor. Do meditation and breathing exercise to combat stress.

Your weight should increase slowly and steadily for the best of your and your baby's health.

During pregnancy, many mothers have craving of some food items which are not healthy if taken in larger amount. This is quite natural in pregnancy due to the first wave of hormones entering in the bloodstream. Usually it is not related with the nutritional deficiency. Pregnancy food cravings fall into a few categories like sweet, spicy, and salty. Some of the common items are chocolates, ice creams, coffee, cakes and cookies, pickles, fried and spicy food, soda, and aerated drinks, etc.

You can have some substitutes to satisfy your cravings. Instead of cake or cookies, you can take toast with the jam.

Instead of fried items, go for the baked food. Fruit juices and coconut water can take place of soda and soft drinks.

Some women have cravings of non-food items such as chalk, clay, crayons, or pencils which are extremely harmful to both mother and baby. This type of condition is called 'Pica'. If you find yourself cravings for any non-food item, consult your doctor and get yourself tested for iron, zinc, or any other nutritional deficiency. Whenever you get cravings, just distract your mind from it. Go for a walk, talk with your friend, or keep yourself busy in some creative activities like in music or reading, which will help you forget about the cravings.

Healthy Habits – Healthy Pregnancy

- Remember the 5 essentials of life: air, water, exercise, sleep, and diet.
- Yoga and exercise in the morning for a better mood and stamina throughout the day.
- Sleep for at least 8 hours a day.
- Take a mid-day break for an hour every day.
- When you have to sit for a long period of time, stand up, walk, or stretch every 20 minutes.
- Limit the use of electronic gadgets and television. Creativity makes your baby genius.
- Be conscious about your posture 24x7. Bad posture in pregnancy will have bad consequences.
- Make your every meal last for at least 20 minutes.
- Avoid refined carbohydrates and simple sugar.

- Plant-based protein is better than animal-based protein. Replace chips, crackers, and snack bars with nuts, fruits, salads, celery.

- Replace sweet and fried foods with healthier spices and flavours to satisfy your cravings.

- Make activity your first line of defence before you resort to painkillers and other medications for your pregnancy discomforts.

- Create a routine so you don't eat, drink, or use electronic messaging in the last hour before you go to bed.

6

The Grand Finale of Pregnancy (Labour and Delivery)

Many of the women, especially in their first pregnancy (primi gravida), have anxiety and fear of labour and childbirth. You might have so many questions in your mind regarding the actual signs of labour, how much will it hurt, how to cope up the pain, and what to do for normal delivery. Don't go by the stories that your mother, sister, or friends have recounted, because as we know, each pregnancy is unique, each labour and childbirth experience can be entirely different. Some labours start with the rhythmic contraction or some may with ruptured membrane. You might have made some birth plans like 'no episiotomy', 'no caesarean', but remember, what happens during your labour is highly unpredictable, so be flexible and sensible and trust your doctor's decision.

The position of your baby's head will determine the type of delivery you will go through.

1. **Occiput anterior:** This is considered to be the easiest position to deliver a baby vaginally. Baby's head is down and facing mother's back. Back of baby's head is facing forward.

2. **Occiput posterior:** Baby's head is down, but back of the head is facing the back of the mother. Here, the baby exerts tremendous pressure on the mother's spine and nerves, which leads to severe back pain. This is sometimes referred as a 'back labour'. In such cases, normal delivery is possible, but labour may take little longer and you are more likely to need an assisted delivery like forceps or episiotomy.

3. **Breech position:** In the uterus, a breech baby is positioned buttocks down (rather than head down) and his head is under your ribs.
   - **Complete breech** – The buttocks are the lowest and legs are crossed and bent at hips and knees.
   - **Frank breech** – Baby is bottom down and legs are straight up bent at hips and straight from the knees. He is facing his own feet. His arms may be around the legs.
   - **Footling breech** – Feet are the lowest. Baby has one or both legs pointing in down position as they are going to come out before the buttocks.

4. **Transverse lie:** In the uterus, the baby lies with its head towards your right or left side, and its buttocks are on the other side.

   Umbilical cord prolapse is a rare but serious complication with breech babies. There might be premature rupture of membrane (bag of water) and umbilical cord falls through the open cervix into vagina before the baby. If the umbilical cord is compressed due to the foetal pressure, then the blood flow to the foetus will be restricted. There might be sudden decrease in the baby's heart rate and it may go into distress. Thus in cases of breech lie or transverse lie, the only safe option is caesarean delivery.

In the 3rd trimester, usually the placenta is placed higher in the uterus. However, if you are detected with '*placenta previa*', which means placenta is lying low in the uterus and close to the cervix, and then your delivery method must be a C-section because any dilation (opening) of cervix will lead to excessive bleeding in case of placenta previa.

GET READY FOR THE CLIMAX

Acquire enough knowledge about the labour and delivery by taking a labour and childbirth class from your antenatal therapist. It would be great if your partner or mother accompany you in your childbirth class so they can learn massage and other comfort measures of labour. In your childbirth class, you can learn about the twists and turns of labour, breathing exercise, comfort measures for pain management, and types of deliveries. During your labour, you may not be able to remember the breathing techniques and positions you have learnt. So at this point, your partner can assist you and make you relax. Once you are familiar and prepared for your big event, your anxiety and fear will be vanished and you become more confident and positive.

In your last month, you and your partner must visit the labour room or maternity unit in your hospital where you are going to deliver your baby. Observe your labour room thoroughly so that you can meditate daily with the focus of the labour room. In your meditation, *'visualize yourself in the labour room. You are in intense pain, but still you are breathing and smiling. No shouting, no crying, and no negative air is allowed here. You are full of energy and stamina. Your soul, your consciousness, is the silent witness of your positivity. You are breathing and pushing, again breathing and pushing and finally giving birth to a beautiful, divine child. He/she is the proof of your existence. He/she is the gift you are giving to this world and nature'.*

If you practise this visualization daily, it will be very effectual in your actual labour and delivery. The childbirth process will go quite smooth and easy both for you and your baby. This is the holistic approach to deliver a baby.

Relaxation Techniques

It is very important to know that stress or fear releases adrenaline hormone (stress hormone) which affects the coordination and functioning of the uterine muscles and thus slows down your labour, while relaxation increases endorphins (body's natural painkiller). So mastering relaxation is your most effective technique for easing labour pain. In the state of relaxation, more oxygen and nutrients travel to both the labouring uterus and to the baby. Even though you may not be able to stay completely relaxed during contractions, your ability to rest and relax between the contractions will increase your stamina and help your body work more efficiently.

Relaxation is a combination of rhythmic breathing and allowing tension to go out of your body. It is an acquired skill which takes time, practise, and patience to develop. So start practising relaxation techniques during your pregnancy only so that it becomes easier for you to relax through it during labour.

Complete Relaxation

- Sit or lie down in your comfortable position using a number of pillows. In late pregnancy, resting flat on your back is not comfortable as well as not advisable. Now start focusing on your body parts one after the other from the toes to your head. First, concentrate on your toes, ankles, and left leg. Feel the heaviness or tightness in the muscles. Breathe in, and as you breathe out, relax your left toes, feet, and ankle muscles completely. Let them roll towards the floor.
- Now focus on your left shin, knee joint, thigh, and hip region. With each exhalation, let go of the tension from these muscles. You can feel your left lower limb very much light and relaxed. In the same way, relax your right lower limb completely.
- Focus on your vagina (birth canal). Tight/squeeze the muscles once and then release it with a relaxing exhalation.
- Now feel the girth of your abdomen. If you feel any tightness in the abdominal muscles, relax them with each exhalation. Relaxed tummy area

will provide more room for your baby. You can feel the movement of your chest as you inhale and exhale. Let your breathing be natural and don't force yourself to inhale or exhale. Feel the complete relaxation from the chest to the toes.

- Next, relax your shoulders, upper arms, elbows, and forearms. Open up your fingers slightly and then release them to be relaxed and loosen completely.

- Release the tension or stress from your neck and back muscles and relax them.

- Shift your focus on your face. Relax all the facial muscles, especially release the tenseness from your forehead, eyebrows, and mouth. Eyes should be closed, but don't force your eyelids to shut the eyes very tightly. Feel the tension draining out of your head.

- Now, once you scan your body, check to see that your whole body is completely relaxed and loose. If you find any tension in any of the muscles, release it now. Feel yourself completely weightless as you are floating in the air.

- Keep inhaling the positivity, energy, and happiness from your surroundings. Throw out your anxiety, fatigue, and aches with each exhalation. In this blissful state of relaxation, connect your consciousness to baby's consciousness. Baby receives all your mental vibrations and enjoys this bonding with you.

- Take your time while coming out of a complete relaxation. Slowly move your fingers and toes, be aware of your surroundings, and open your eyes. You will enjoy this relaxation much more if your partner or antenatal therapist guides you throughout the relaxation in a slow and soothing voice.

Roving Body Check (Touch Relaxation)

Partner plays a crucial role during labour, especially a light touch and a soothing voice of a husband can pamper you and help you to be relaxed. It is wonderful if partner can figure out where you are holding tension. You will often tense up your forehead, eyebrows, and jaw during labour. Husband can rest his hands or can stroke lightly where you are holding tension. This is the most effective and encouraging for the mother to relax that part. Further, most of the women hold tension in the shoulders and hands as you make a tight fist or you hold something very tightly during painful contractions. Here, husband can pat his hand soothingly over your arms and hands. Sometimes in the intense pain, mom wants her husband to squeeze her hand which in turns helps her to reduce the tension.

During your labour, in between the contractions, this kind of roving and relaxing is very much remedial and adaptable for the well-off progress of labour.

Get Ready for the Hospital

A checklist of what you should pack for your delivery. Ensure you have packed your hospital bag before you reach full term, or you will be in rush if your little one decides to arrive early.

1. Medical records – so they are ready for your doctor.
2. Long T-shirt or short gown to wear in labour.
3. Socks – because your feet get cold in labour.
4. Extra pillows – for comfort during and after labour.
5. Aromatherapy oils/candles to help you relax.
6. Feeding pillow.
7. Sweets to suck for energy during labour.
8. Cold water spray for your face, especially in hot hospital rooms.
9. Juice, energy drink, or lemonade to quench thirst and for energy.
10. Hot water bottle or ice packs to help relieve pain.
11. Thick sanitary napkins for post-delivery usage.
12. Toiletries to freshen up.
13. Nightgown with buttons for easy feeding access.
14. Nursing or front-opening bra and breast pads.
15. Nipple cream to avoid cracking.
16. Nappies/diapers for the newborn.
17. 5 baby outfits, vests, and socks for the newborn.
18. Nappy rash cream – just in case.
19. Baby's oil and body wash for bath.
20. Breast pump – if required.
21. Slippers.

Learn to Overcome Your Fears

Many of the women spend their whole pregnancy worrying about their negative thoughts and weaknesses to accomplish their upcoming responsibilities. But what is the gain from this kind of anxiety, better you develop yourself mentally and emotionally to combat your future challenges.

Fear

- I will not be able to make it through labour and delivery.
- I will not be able to take good care of my baby once it arrives.
- I am not capable to deal with the new challenges and responsibilities.
- I will never gain my pre-pregnancy figure and charm back. My career will be finished.

Faith

- I will have the inner strength and help I need to have a good birth experience.
- I am going to educate myself by available resources and I will enjoy my motherhood.
- I have confidence in myself and I will bring about the best I can. I will ask for help when I need it.
- I will definitely take time for myself. I have resolved that I shall live to the fullest.

Make a chart of your inner fear and faith and stick this on the wall of your room. Initially read both the aspects, but the faith should be read aloud. Keep reminding yourself that you have to convert your fear into the faith. Gradually as you feel your fear has abbreviated, then only faith should be there—on the wall and in your mind.

Read your faiths daily. The most rewarding benefit of this mental activity is that with practise you can throw away the negativity and concentrate on the positives. Your baby receives and understands most of your feelings and emotions. If you want your baby to be happy and optimist, first work on yourself. Your positive attitude will nurture baby's inner environment.

PRELUDE TO LABOUR (Labour Signs)

Some few days or may be few hours before your labour, you may experience some of the following signs and symptoms. But these signs may be variable in every individual.

- *Lightning sensation:* In the last month, as you are approaching your due date, the baby drops lower in the pelvis and settles in a headlock position. As the baby sinks down, the pressure from the ribs will be released. Your breathing and eating become easier. But the pelvic pressure and frequency of urination will be increased.

- *Nesting instinct:* Not all the women experience it. But some of you in the last weeks of pregnancy feel yourself full of stamina and energy and urge to clean and organise your house before the baby arrives. This is because the large amount of adrenaline is released in your body. It's just nature's way to make you ready for the big event. So take advantage of this energy booster and complete your pending works. Remember, do not overexert yourself now and conserve some energy for the strenuous process of labour and delivery.

- *Gastric discomfort:* Many of the women have a sensation of vomiting and diarrhoea as a beginning of the labour. During the early part of labour, the body needs to release prostaglandin hormones to start uterine contraction. This hormone over-stimulates your bowel and leads to frequent stools.

- *Braxton Hicks contraction:* These are the false pains that confuse you about the true labour. The contractions are arrhythmic, irregular, and mostly painless, but sometimes uncomfortable. Unlike true labour, they do not increase in frequency and intensity and then stop suddenly or vanish with walking, eating, drinking, or changing activity/position.

- *Cervical effacement:* Cervix is the area between uterus and vagina. The normal cervix is generally 1–2 inches (2–5 cm) long and quite firm. Due to prostaglandin hormones, cervix prepares itself for delivery and it becomes soft and riper. The process when ripe cervix gradually becomes thinner and shorter is called effacement. The cervix must be 100% effaced or paper thin before it begins to dilate or open. At this stage, you will be going into labour in no time (Fig. 6.1).

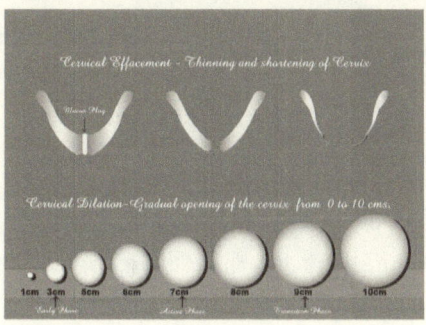

- ***Mucus plug discharge:*** In pregnancy, the mucus plug is like a tight seal on the cervix between your vagina and uterus. It blocks the way for any bacteria or fungal infection from the vagina to the uterus, and thus protecting your baby. Now as the effacement process occurs and cervix begins to thin and ripe, it loosens the mucus plug and dislodges it. It looks like a thick blood-tinged jelly or mucus. You may notice this reddish brown discharge while urinating or bathing or in your panties. It may go unnoticed sometimes. Losing your mucus plug indicates that your labour is on its way.

- ***Breaking the water:*** It is also called rupture of the membrane (amniotic sac). Once your mucus plug is dropped, the amniotic sac can rupture anytime. A hole or tear in the water bag (amniotic sac) leads to a dribbling or a gush of discharge. You may think you are urinating, but you will find that you are not able to control it. In such case, contact your doctor immediately or go to the hospital. You will probably go into labour within 12–24 hours. Usually the colour of this fluid is clear or slightly pink. If it is yellowish green, it might be strained with the meconium (baby's stool) and leads to foetal distress.

STAGES OF LABOUR AND DELIVERY

The Exciting 'Labour Day' Has Come

Labour is undoubtedly a physical and emotional marathon, so it is wise to approach labour with the proper understanding that it has three main stages. The pain you feel is actually the uterine muscle contractions. Muscles of the uterus tighten and relax during contractions. You feel the pain/contractions as a severe discomfort, menstrual-like cramps, or as a persistent backache.

Stage I

First stage starts with the onset of contractions and lasts until your cervix has dilated fully (10 cm) from which baby's head is able to pass through. This is the longest stage. Average duration of 1st stage is 12–16 hours for primi gravida (woman with 1st delivery) and 6–8 hours in multipara (woman with one or more deliveries in the past). This stage is further divided into three phases called early, active, and transition phase.

- *Early (latent) phase:* This is the longest among the three phases, lasting for 8–10 hours (considering primi gravida). Herein cervix opens from 0 to 3 cm. Short and light contractions come at 10–15 minutes interval and last for 15–20 seconds each time. If your bag of water has not broken before the onset of labour, it ruptures during labour with the force of contractions. Some women may not even notice this stage initially as the contractions are just uncomfortable, not painful. You may be excited and positive at this stage.

- *Active phase:* You may notice that it takes some efforts to get through the contractions as you go from the early phase to active phase of labour. Contractions are getting longer, stronger, and closer together. They last for 40–60 seconds and come at every 3–4 minutes apart. Active phase lasts for about

4–5 hours. At this phase, cervix opens or dilates about 7 cm. On average, your cervix will dilate at approximately 1 cm/hr. About 25% of women experience back labour at this phase. Normally when labour begins, the baby is in Occiput-anterior position, which means it is facing the mother's back. This is the easiest position for vaginal delivery. But if baby is settled in the Occiput-posterior position, then the hard back of baby's skull puts pressure on mother's backbone. This leads to severe discomfort and pain in your lower back and between your buttocks. As this phase progresses, you may lose your appetite and start to feel sick. You cannot walk and talk through each contraction. You may need to stop moving, working, or whatever you are doing and just sit down during contractions. This is the time you should leave for the hospital.

- **_Transition phase:_** This is the shortest but the toughest phase amongst all. It lasts for 30 minutes to 2 hours. You get erratic and hard contractions now at an interval of 1–2 minutes and last for 90 seconds. The cervix dilates between 8 and 10 cm. You may feel pressure on the perineum (space between vagina and rectum) as the baby's head descends further in the birth canal. So you get the urge to bear down (push). But if your cervix is not fully dilated, i.e., 10 cm, you are not supposed to push, otherwise you will damage your cervix and baby's head. Feeling agitated, crying, experiencing nausea, vomiting, sweating, coldness, shaking, rectal pressure are the normal symptoms at this phase.

Stage II

This is the pushing and delivery stage. Duration of 2nd stage of labour is anywhere between 20 minutes to 2 hours. Contractions are more expulsive but less intense than transition phase. They come at an interval of 3–5 minutes and last for 60–90 seconds. Your cervix is completely dilated, so now you are shifted to the labour room. You will be given the pushing position on a delivery couch (Fig.6.2). The most common position used for pushing is semi-reclined position. The head of your bed is elevated to 45°. Your legs should be wide apart and bent from your knees. You must have a strong natural urge to push. Now once your doctor says, you can bear down using all your energy. With each contraction, baby moves closer to the opening of the birth canal. As you bear down with controlled breathing, gradually the head of the baby begins to appear. Sometimes the head slips back between the contractions, but eventually it comes out of vagina (just like your head emerges out from the polo neck T-shirt). This is called crowning. At this point, you should breathe slowly and don't push hard as it may damage the perineum tissues. You will feel hot and burning sensations around your perineum, and this condition is being known as the 'ring of fire'. Baby's head is delivered facing the floor and then the baby rotates to one of the sides. The next contraction and your pushing efforts will deliver its shoulders. Then the rest of body will slip out easily, with the gush of

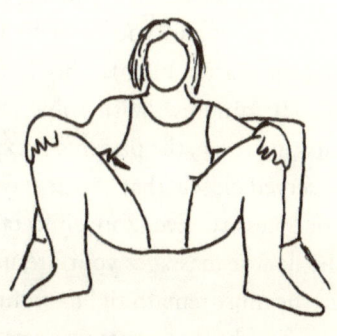

amniotic fluid and sometimes some blood too. Doctor will then suck out mucus or amniotic fluid from baby's nose and mouth with a bulb syringe. Now baby can take its first breath and begin to cry. Umbilical cord will be cut and clamped.

Stage III

Congratulations, you have done it. Your tough time is over now and you enter in the stage 3, i.e., delivery of placenta (after birth). This is the shortage stage of about 10–20 minutes. With some labour-like contractions and pushing force, the placenta is expelled out easily. You will be observed closely that uterus stays contracted and bleeding is not excessive. Even some injectable medicines are given, and the doctor massages your uterus until it becomes firm. The uterus must remain tight and firm to prevent bleeding from the site where placenta was attached to the wall of uterus.

How To Make Your Labour Easy

Herein partner plays a very important role in labour. Labour and childbirth is a stressful and tiring period for soon-to-be mother. At this point, partner can be a great source of strength and support to her. During labour, you are the first person she looks to for help. During labour, she might forget what she's supposed to do, so this is your time to remind her about the breathing and apply all the skills and tips you have learnt in your childbirth class. Similarly, you are developing a strong bond with your unborn child. Medical research indicates that women who go through labour with their husband coaching them have a more positive experience and often a shorter labour.

Labour Breathing

At rest, our breathing is slow and rhythmic, but when we are tensed, automatically our breathing becomes erratic or we may hold our breath, so it is very important to learn controlled breathing in labour. Just reading about and understanding labour breathing will not be helpful at all. You need to practise this 'Lamaze breathing' daily that you have learnt in your labour class. Then and then you will be able to work on it and get benefited from it during labour. Breathing should become an automatic response to pain. Labour period is just like an exam. You have to start preparation well in advance to get good result.

Your natural, controlled, and rhythmic breathing that goes on with contractions/pain helps you in many ways.

a) It keeps your body filled with the energy necessary for its hard work.

b) It increases the oxygen supply to the muscles and thus allows the body to work effectively with contractions.

c) You can provide more oxygen to your baby too.

d) Breathing will overcome your urge to push if it is not the right time to push.

e) The focal point on which you are focusing while breathing will divert your mind and fix your awareness. Concentration on any inner or outer focal point is beneficial for easing you through each contraction and reducing your pain perception. Relaxation techniques along with the breathing will reduce the chances of assisted birth.

Different Patterns of Breathing Are Used at Different Phases

1. **Deep cleansing and relaxing breath:** Sit in your comfortable position. Take a slow and deep inhalation through the nose to the count of 6. Then exhale slowly through the mouth to the count of 6 and release all the tension from the body. Remember, do not let the in-breath become longer than the out-breath. Vice versa will be fine. Deep cleansing breath should be done in each phase (early, active, and transition) of stage 1 labour at the beginning and at the end of each contractions/pain. This breathing helps to sharpen your focus and provide more oxygen to your baby and your uterus.

2. **Slow pursed lip breathing (early labour breathing):** This breathing is used in early phase of labour when your contractions are mild and 15 minutes apart. As your pain starts, take one deep cleansing breath first. Then inhale to a count of 4 and exhale through pursed lips as if you were whistling, counting 4 in your mind. Keep your eyes open if you are using outside focal point. If you find it relaxing, there is nothing wrong in making a sound on the out breath like "oooh . . ." or "aaahhh . . ." Repeat this breathing throughout your pain. Once your pain stops, take one or two

deep cleansing breath and then enjoy the pain-free period.

3. **Light breath for mid labour:** This should be done in the active phase of labour, when the contractions are intense and you cannot walk or talk through your pain. As your contraction grows, your breathing rate should be increased and you should be more focused and alert to cope up. At this point, if you become tense or panic, you will start over breathing which may lead to hyperventilation. As a result, you may feel dizziness and lightheaded. Some women make their body tight and hold their breaths, which will reduce the oxygen supply to you and your baby, so it is very important to learn and practise the focused and controlled breathing. Now as you enter in an active phase where your pain lasts for 40–60 seconds and comes at every 3–4 minutes, you have to start light breathing. First, take a deep cleansing breath. Now take a shallow inhalation through your nose or mouth to a count of 2 and then exhalation through mouth in a count of 2. Continue it throughout your pain. Your inhalation should be quiet, but exhalation can be audible. When your contraction ends, take a couple of deep relaxing breath.

4. **Pant-pant-blow (hee-hee-hoo) breathing:** In transition phase, as your contraction starts, take a deep cleansing breath (count of 6) and letting go of all the tension from the body as you breathe out. Now focus your attention on the focal point, it may either be your partner's face or any picture

on the wall. Inhale through your nose preferably, and then exhale in two short pants, thus create a rhythmic pattern. Keep your facial muscles relaxed; continue this breathing until the contractions stop. End with a deep relaxing breath. In short, you can use 1 in-breath and 2 out-breaths or 2 shallow in-breaths and one long out-breath. Practise both the breathings and choose one for labour. During the contractions, you may have a strong urge to push the baby out, but you are not supposed to do that as your cervix is not completely open yet. So in this situation, use a blowing breath. Inhale and puff your cheeks out and blow out the air with force as if you are blowing several candles at a time. This diminishes your pushing urge until the proper time.

5. **Pushing breath:** Your urge to push comes with each contraction. It feels like being very constipated and having a bowel movement just now to get relief. You will be given the pushing position in the labour room. As your contraction comes, take one deep cleansing breath. Then take one deep inhalation and push with all of your might, while making your abdominal muscles tight and while holding your breath to the count of 10 (your nurse or partner will guide you by counting). After 10 seconds, release your breath. Continue this pattern: inhale, hold your breath and push, and exhale until the contractions go away. The latest research indicates that holding your breath while pushing goes against the body's natural desire to push, and sometimes baby may not tolerate your breath hold. So the 'controlled exhalation breathing' works better

for some women. In this pattern, after a deep inhalation, rather than holding your breath while pushing let air slowly escape through your pursed lips. Keep your abdominal muscles tight during pushing. Making grunting or moaning sounds, which sometimes come naturally, help women to release tension. After 8–10 seconds, release your breath completely. Repeat the pattern throughout your contraction. With controlled exhalation breathing, you gently ease your baby down and out. Thus you can avoid episiotomy and prevent your perineum from tearing. Your doctor may tell you stop pushing and blow for a couple of contractions just to regain some strength and keep the baby to be born too quickly.

Be Active In Between the Contractions

Above-mentioned breathing exercises are to be done during the contractions (pain). Once your pain stops and you enter in the pain-free period, don't just confine yourself to the bed. The more you are moving and staying in the upright postures (positions), the faster and easier your labour will be. Walking or moving around is the perfect tool for the pain management. Gravitational force will help the baby to descend and thus reduce the labour time and fasten the delivery. Studies show that women who were encouraged to walk or change positions during labour tend to have shorter labour, more efficient contractions, greater comfort, and least requirements for painless or assisted delivery. Adopt the positions, which tilt your torso forward, and thus utilise the force of gravity to help in pushing and birth process along. Because of the ante-version of the uterus during 1st stage contractions, many women find that they instinctively need to lean forward on some sort of support. Some women like to rotate or rock their pelvis. Women should be encouraged to change positions during the first stage of labour. The different postures that you would like to use during labour are demonstrated here. Partners should also be aware of these postures, because sometimes you become so overwhelmed and frightened to move. At this point, your partner is the one who can suggest and help you in adopting the alternatives.

- Forward lean on ball or on a back of armless chair (Fig. 6.3)

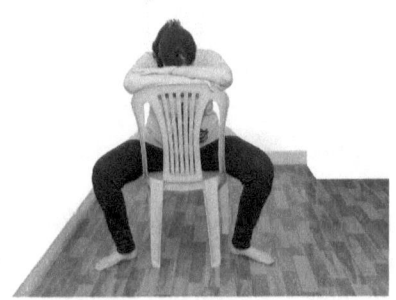

- Lunge position (Fig. 6.4)

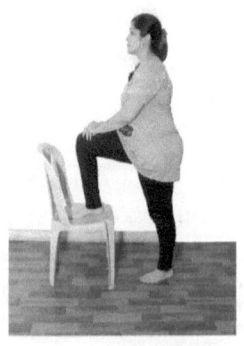

- Cat and camel position
- Walking around (if you are not tired)
- Squatting while holding some support
- Cross-leg sitting with back support
- Side lying position with couple of pillows for comfort
- Semi-reclining position

Massage

Before the advent of the use of anaesthesia during labour in the mid nineteenth century, massage was widely used to provide general sense of well-being and relax the labouring body. Research showed that women who were massaged by partner during labour were less anxious, suffered less pain, had shorter labour, had greater ability to cope, and were less likely to suffer from postnatal depression.

- Use scented oil like lavender, chamomile, or ylang ylang for massage to reduce friction and enhancing the relaxation. You will also get the benefit of aromatherapy here.
- Use long flowing strokes either using your whole palms or just finger tips for back. Your strokes should be slow, rhythmic, longitudinal, pleasant, or according to her need. Avoid massaging over the spine (backbone).
- Pain is most commonly experienced over the lower half of the abdomen. So light finger stroking or brushing (pampering with the hands) over the pain region from one side to the other is often well appreciated. Deep massage is totally unacceptable. Women often spontaneously start rubbing their

abdomen themselves. It should be encouraged if it is helpful to you.

- Provide firm circular pressure and mild squeezing to the shoulder and shoulder blade muscles. This can help you to relax your shoulders and breathe rhythmically.
- Sometimes feet become very cold in labour. So firm strokes from ankle to toes and circular massage over the soles will help to warm them up. Effleurage or kneading over the calf muscles will relieve the cramps.
- If you are given epidural in case of painless labour, you can't feel any sensation on your back and feet. So hand massage is ideal here. Gently pull each finger in turn to release tension. Simple strokes on the palm and on the back of hands will be very soothing.
- Light brushing strokes with fingers over the forehead and face will relieve tension from the facial muscles.

OTHER COMFORT MEASURES

1. Hot packs to lower abdomen, to groin, or to perineum will relieve the pain.
2. Cold packs can be applied to lower back. Be careful not to burn or freeze the skin through prolonged exposure.
3. Mental activities like chanting, counting breaths, and imagination (visualisation) is often well received.
4. Music therapy – Soft and quiet relaxation music will enhance your relaxation. The music that you

have heard throughout your prenatal period will definitely work for you in your labour. Familiar music can help you to calm, provide comfort, and help to focus on breathing. It decreases the need for the analgesic medication during birth and contributes to overall positive feelings about the birth process.

5. For back labour: When your baby is in posterior position, which means back of baby's head is against the mother's tailbone, you are likely to get a great amount of pressure and pain in your lower back during and between the contractions. In this case, crawling position (on your hands and knee position), forward bending, or lunge position may give you some comforts.

    ▪ Your partner can do a 'double hip squeeze' by putting his hands on the back of your hips and squeezing together towards your tailbone.

    ▪ 'Knee press' or 'counter pressure' are also good measures to get pain relief, which can be done by your partner.

Labour Tips

Early Phase

▪ Contractions last for 15–20 seconds and come after every 10–15 minutes.
▪ Keep moving normally.
▪ Do abdominal breathing or slow pursed lip breathing of early phase.

- Some women describe first sign of labour as a discomfort, not much painful, while others find the pain is difficult to cope with.

- If pains are only uncomfortable and lack of intensity, you can continue with your normal activity. Take a walk, but not to the point of exhaustion. Take rest in between as you have a long way to go. When you feel contractions are more intense, it's time to go to the hospital.

- Your mother or grandmother may offer you a glass of milk or sweet preparations before going to the hospital for delivery. Their intension must be to provide you with the energy for labour and delivery. But it is not advisable to take heavy food once your labour starts. If you feel weakness or feel like eating something, take some light snacks or fruit juice for energy. If you eat heavy things like ghee, almond milk, or sweets during labour, you might feel nausea or vomiting. With other aspects, if you have to go for C-section for any reason, you are required to be on an empty stomach.

- Use the breathing and comfort positions for early phase. Staying active in the early phase encourage your cervix to dilate more quickly. But don't exhaust yourself.

- It is normal to feel anxious at hospital environment, but be relaxed. Fear or tension may slow down your labour.

- Stay positive and just tell yourself that you are going to welcome your baby very soon.

Dad's Job

- Your role as a birth partner is vital.
- Encourage her to move, but don't get her tired.
- Give her sweet drinks and light snacks.
- Remind her to empty her bladder frequently because full bladder will restrict the space for uterus to contract and thus slow down the labour. Even the baby's presenting part (usually the head) presses firmly against the bladder and bowel as he descends through the pelvis. This can lead to an intense pain particularly if mother's bladder is full.
- Help her to get comfort by a number of pillows, giving massage, light music therapy, and aromatherapy.
- You can even breathe with her if she can't cope with contractions.
- If labour is slow, help her to change the mood and surroundings. Take her for a walk or move her to another room. Talk with her about your sweet memories.
- Be encouraging and don't hurry her.
- Even you also require some food and drinks to keep up your energy. If you are drained, you can't help her.

Active Phase

- Contractions last for 40–60 seconds and come at an interval of 3–4 minutes.
- In this phase, between the contractions, change your positions frequently like sitting, and leaning on the back of a chair, hold a hug position to your

partner, zen position (vajrasana) with the knees open and head resting forward on the ball, bean bag, or chair.

- Do light breathing.
- Urinate frequently.
- During active phase, staircase climbing, hip rocking exercise, or slow dancing with your partner will be very beneficial. The swaying movements of hips guide the baby into the pelvic opening and help the baby move into the optimal position for birth.

Transition Phase

- Contractions last for 90 seconds and come at every 60–90 seconds.
- Do pant-pant-blow breathing.
- Between contractions, keep changing your positions like kneeling, crawling (cat and camel), leaning forward on your partner, or on a wall, semi-sitting or semi-reclining position with number of pillows for comfort.
- You may feel distressed, exhausted, or may be out of control as you are at the hardest point of labour. Some women may feel sick or get mild diarrhoea. If you have backache, moving your hips in a circular motion (belly dancing) will give you some relief. Massage will be helpful.
- If you are tired, lie down on your one side or even better rest forward on the side of bed or bean bag or ball. Do not lie on your back. Squatting or just being upright helps in dilatation.

- Don't worry about what people will think, do what you need to do. You may want to be alone with your partner only.

Dad's Job

- Accept and understand her tears and mood. You keep yourself calm.
- Pamper her as much as possible with your hands, eyes, voice, and reassuring presence.
- Create more privacy and keep disturbance to minimum.
- Make sure that she keeps her body relaxed and loose. Take care she is not clinching her teeth.
- Give her some drink or ice to suck.
- Give her relaxing massage. Apply rolling pin or wet towel for backache.
- Remind her to do blowing breathing if she has urge to push at this phase.

Pushing Stage

- The most common position for pushing is in semi-sitting reclining position with legs wide apart and bent from knees. During contractions, place your hands underneath your knees to facilitate pushing.
- Making loud sounds while releasing your breath will help you be relaxed.

Dad's Job

- Encourage her to push only when she needs to push.

- Give her sweet juice or drinks to maintain her energy level.
- Keep reminding her to relax her face, especially jaws and teeth.
- Remind her the pushing breath and make deep 'aaah . . .' sounds with her.

During Contraction (Normal Labour)

Mom

- Phase-related breathing exercise
- Self-effleurage (massage) on abdomen
- Chanting

Dad

- Breathing exercise
- Encourage her
- Visualisation

Between Contraction (Normal Labour)

Mom

- Changing position
- Walking
- Relaxation
- Climbing stairs

Dad

- Hand/foot massage

- Back massage
- Aromatherapy (camomile, lavender, sandalwood)
- Music therapy (Sitar, Santoor, Omkar)

During Contraction (Back Labour)

Mom

- Phase-related breathing
- Self-effleurage

Dad

- Counter pressure
- Double hip squeeze
- Knee press
- Ice pack application
- Encouragement

Between Contractions (Back Labour)

Mom

- Pelvic rocking
- Lunge position
- Walking
- Changing position

Dad

- Ice pack application
- Back massage
- Music and aromatherapy

Baby Is Born!

Congratulations! Your long-awaited bundle of joy is here. Take your time to enjoy your baby's presence because the first few moments are vital for bonding. You may be feeling the roller-coaster ride of emotions. Tears of happiness and excitement come with the state of apprehension and uncertainty. This happens to each and every mother.

Dad's Job

- After placenta is removed, if you want, you can cut the umbilical cord. This is quite an emotional moment for dad.
- Your physical and emotional support is very essential for the new mother's well-being and good recovery. Her body has gone through tremendous amount of stress in the last few days. Her hormones are also dropping suddenly, so you need to understand her psychological stress and mood swings.
- Enjoy your life's one of the best and precious moments as a family.

Assisted Labour and Delivery

Epidural (Painless Labour)

Pain is the synonym of labour. All the mothers-to-be have different pain threshold and react differently to their labour pain. Some may be able to cope with it, while for others it is immeasurable. But now it is possible to have a normal delivery without the pain—by the use of an 'epidural'. It is the regional anaesthesia and most effective form of pain relief, which works in more than 90% of cases. Once your labour has started, you can request for an epidural at any point of time.

An anaesthetist will insert a small flexible tube into the base of the spine (in lumber region) through which the drug is injected. This medical procedure will take about 10–30 minutes to complete. The nerves that carry pain sensations is blocked at spinal level and not allowed to reach to brain. Within 20 minutes, you feel complete numbness in the lower abdomen, birth canal, and legs (whole lower body). You will probably no longer feel contractions now. You need to be monitored constantly by an anaesthetist. Although epidural anaesthesia is safe and does not affect your baby, you should be aware about some side effects and disadvantages of it.

- Your movement is severely or totally restricted. You have to be in bed until the baby is born. 'Walking epidurals' may allow some mobility.
- Epidural anaesthesia will cease your sensations down the waist. You will not get sensations even if your bladder is full, so you may need to be catheterised.
- Epidural interfere with all of the labour hormones, so it can slow down the contractions or may stop the labour. A drip might be needed to speed up the things.
- Mother cannot feel contractions, so pushing may be more difficult.
- The most common side effect of epidural is hypotension (drop in maternal blood pressure).
- Other consequences of epidural are nausea, itching, and/or fever, if medication lasts for more than 6 hours.

- Many women complain of mild pain and tenderness postpartum at the epidural site.

Episiotomy

As the baby's head comes through the opening of the vagina (which is called crowning), the skin and muscles of vagina and perineum are being stretched. There are chances of inappropriate tearing of the delicate tissues. Episiotomy is a small incision made in the perineum from the vagina towards the anus. This will widen the passage and facilitate the easy delivery. Your doctor will recommend episiotomy when,

- there is a risk of extensive vaginal tearing,
- your baby is large or baby is in abnormal position, or
- baby needs to be delivered quickly.

You will be given local anaesthesia to numb the tissues so you will not feel the cut. The incision may be middle or mediolateral. After delivery, doctor will stitch the incision. You can use ice packs over your perineum to reduce the pain and swelling. These stitches should be dissolved within 15–20 days.

Forceps Birth

When the mother is exhausted and needs assistance or unable to push (may be due to epidural), forceps method is used to deliver a baby. It is also used when there is sudden foetal distress and baby's head is low enough in the pelvis. At this point, baby needs to be delivered vaginally more safely and quickly than a C-section. Forceps are a pair of smooth, metal instrument that has a handle at one end and the other end has 2 curves (spoons) that can cradle baby's head.

The doctor will put an episiotomy. Then the forceps are gently inserted into the vagina one at a time to each side of your baby's head. Turning the forceps can turn the baby's head into an occipito-anterior position and thus facilitate the delivery. With each contraction and with your pushing force, doctor will gently pull the forceps and thus pull out the baby through vagina. Sometimes baby is born with some red marks or bruises over the cheeks. These are the temporary forceps marks and will clear up within a few days.

Vacuum/Ventouse

This is an alternative to forceps delivery. Indications for the vacuum delivery are the same as those for the forceps. The choice between forceps or vacuum may depend on which is the most appropriate in the particular situation. In vacuum-assisted delivery, a soft funnel-shaped plastic cup or a rigid (firm) mushroom-shaped metal cup is used. This cup is placed on the top of baby's scalp. A vacuum is generated inside the cup with a special suction device so that the cup is attached firmly to the baby's head. While you push with each contraction, the doctor gently pull the cup like in forceps and guide the baby down the birth canal.

Babies who are born by vacuum-assisted delivery might have mild swelling and bruising over the back of their head where the vacuum cup has been placed. This usually resolves on its own within hours or days.

Caesarean Delivery (C-section)

Nowadays, C-section operations are being more common and acceptable. Doctors' training and consents towards forceps and vacuum have been decreased. Your C-section may be either pre-planned (elective) or as an emergency caesarean. Doctor recommends you a C-section when vagina delivery is unsafe for you and your baby.

1) Indications for a Planned Caesarean: The risk of respiratory distress is higher in babies born by premature caesarean section. Therefore, planned C-section should not be routinely carried out before 36 weeks. There are some reasons that a caesarean section may be planned before labour signs begin:
   - Position of the baby: If baby is in breech position or lying horizontally and does not turn to head down position till end, you will be advised to go for a C-section as it reduces the morbidity for mother and baby.
   - Multiple pregnancies: If you are carrying twins or triplets.
   - Placenta previa: If placenta partially or completely covers the cervix, then delivery should be a planned caesarean.
   - Cervical tumour, any maternal infections or illness like severe pre-eclampsia where mother cannot tolerate a vaginal delivery.
   - A previous C-section or any other surgery on uterus.
   - Maternal request.

2) Indications for Emergency Caesarean: During labour, if doctor suspects any danger to the mother' or baby's condition, an emergency C-section is directed to.

- Foetal morbidity: If the baby's heart rate becomes slow or irregular, it indicates that baby is getting less oxygen and not tolerating labour anymore. If the baby has passed meconium (stool), it is considered to be an emergency and the baby has to be delivered immediately.

- Prolapsed cord occurs when the umbilical cord moves ahead of the baby in vagina. The cord can be compressed and trapped against the baby's body during delivery. This can result in a loss of oxygen to the foetus. Considering it as a danger to the baby, immediate C-section will be performed. Umbilical cord prolapse occurs one in every 300 births.

- Dystocia: Abnormal progress of labour or it does not progress at all. Either the cervix does not dilate or baby's head does not descend to allow vaginal delivery. This has most commonly happened with the drugs used for induction of labour.

- Cephalo pelvic disproportion (CPD): 'Cephalo' means 'baby's head'. Sometimes the baby's head is larger or mother's pelvis is smaller or misshapen that does not allow baby's head to pass through. This can be identified once the labour has started and even with the normal contractions and good pushing efforts, baby is not able to descend in the pelvis.

With the advanced antibiotics, anaesthesia, and surgical technologies, the C-section has become quite safe and very less painful procedure. In this surgery, you will have 2 incisions: one the abdominal skin and the other in your uterus. Usually a spinal anaesthesia or an epidural is given to keep you awake during the operation. In spinal block, your lower body (from the nipple line down to the toes) becomes numb, but you are completely aware about what's going on in the operation theatre.

A small horizontal cut is made in your abdominal skin slight above the pubic hair line. This is also called a 'bikini incision'. After opening and separating the tissues and muscles inside, the doctor will make a second cut in the lower section of the uterus. You might have heard the operation is sometimes called a 'lower segment caesarean section' (LSCS).

Stitches on your abdominal skin may be painful for the initial few days. Your internal stitches will get dissolved themselves and the external sutures are removed on the eighth day. In all caesarean sections, there is a very small risk of trauma or injury to the baby or a foetal breathing problem. Blood loss or bleeding is generally more in the C-section delivery than in the normal delivery. Wound infection or injury to the other organs is the risk associated with any kind of surgery. Despite being safe and common, you need to have enough rest and support after C-section delivery.

- You should avoid lifting, driving, and some household work for initial 7–8 weeks.
- Numbness and/or pain around the incision site are common side effects with the C-section. This happens due to injury to the nerves at the time of surgery.
- Learn and adopt different positions for breastfeeding and for carrying your baby.

7

Pregnancy Jet Lag

POSTPARTUM CHANGES AND CARE

After delivery, until the mother's body has recovered and nearly returned to its pre-pregnant state, it is the postnatal period. It usually lasts 5–6 weeks for normal delivery and 8–10 weeks for caesarean delivery.

As all the pregnancy and labour hormones come down, you will be progressing through many physical and emotional changes. You need to take good care of yourself to deal with all the changes and to rebuild your strength. You have to learn and adopt some adjustments required to fulfil your new role of motherhood.

Immediately after delivery, you will lose 5–6 kg of weight. With the proper diet plan and regular exercise program, you will get your pre-pregnant weight by 10–12 months postpartum.

By 6 weeks postpartum, the uterus shrinks and comes to its original size and weight (80 g). It continues to contract even after delivery to control the excessive bleeding. That is the reason many new mothers feel lower abdominal pain called '*after-birth pains*'. These are more noticeable during breastfeeding because nipple stimulation leads to oxytocin hormone release, which in turn contracts the uterus. You can apply hot packs to abdomen to relieve the discomfort. Physiotherapy exercise, oral analgesic, change in positions, and frequent urination will be helpful in after-birth pains. Whenever these pains are severe, transcutaneous electrical nerve stimulation (TENS) therapy is also given. The therapist uses a small machine that gives low voltage electrical current for pain relief.

As a part of healing process after any kind of delivery, you will have a heavy vaginal bleeding for the initial 3–5 days. This is called '*Lochia*' and it consists of blood from the uterine wall to where the placenta was attached and mucus and blood from the healing cervix. After a few days, the bleeding will decrease in amount and colour changes from red to pinkish brown and finally to pale yellow (watery consistency). To avoid infection, clean your vagina frequently and change your pads as and when required depending on your bleeding (at least every 3 hours). Never use tampons as your body is still healing and tampons could potentially cause trauma. Bleeding lasts for 3–6 weeks in most of the mothers. If you have very heavy bleeding, foul-smelling

Lochia with lots of large blood clots, then immediately call your doctor without ignoring it.

Perineum muscle strength will regain after 5–6 weeks of delivery. Take care of your episiotomy if it is done. Keep a few sterile cotton swabs in a bowl containing antiseptic liquid diluted with water. Every time you go to the toilet, clean your stitches and surrounding area with the swab and gently dry it with a gauze piece. Apply antiseptic cream over the stitches and place a rectangular piece of sterile gauze over it. Cover it with a sanitary napkin and wear a well-fitted panty to keep a pad in place. Your stitches will dissolve in 8–10 days. Use ice packs over perineum for comfort and pain relief. Kegel exercise (pelvic floor strengthening), proper nutrition, and hygiene will fasten your recovery. In case of episiotomy or caesarean, you will get stretching pain over stitches while coughing or sneezing. So support your stitches with hands and lean forward while you laugh or cough. Women must be helped to experiment to find comfortable positioning for feeding, relaxation, and sleep, using pillows or a foam rubber ring. Pain relief can occur rapidly if the mother's weight is advantageously redistributed.

In the breastfeeding mothers, your monthly periods may not return for several months. The hormones needed to produce breast milk (prolactin) can suppress the reproductive hormones. Therefore, your body does not release an egg and you most likely would not menstruate. However, if you are not breastfeeding, resumption of your period will be within 7–9 weeks after delivery. Every woman's body and circumstances are different, so no one can predict exactly when you will get your first postpartum period. Your initial periods after delivery might be irregular and different than before as your body is recovering and readjusting. You might suffer from cramps and blood clots.

In the normal delivery, the vagina was stretched enough to allow the delivery of the baby. It will take about 3–4 weeks to come back in the normal size.

You can have sex after 6 weeks once your episiotomy/C-section wound and vagina are healed, Lochia have ceased, and you are physically and emotionally comfortable. You might be facing dramatic changes in yourself in terms of low libido, vaginal dryness due to decreasing level of oestrogen hormone, adjusting to stressful motherhood, lack of confidence due to body shape, fatigue, etc. These are the reasons you may not feel like having sex. Take it easy and normal. Talk to your partner and let him know what feels good and what does not without forcing yourself into lovemaking.

Consult and discuss with your gynaecologist about the birth control. You may get pregnant again even if you breastfeed your baby and even before you get your first period after delivery, so it is advisable to use any of the contraceptives methods.

Caring Yourself

Any kind of physical exertion should be avoided. As and when you get time, sleep and rest yourself because a new mother may get exhausted and frustrated with the sudden load of responsibilities. You are likely to need several 'rest and relaxation' session daily during the early weeks. New mothers should be asked for help with their household chores and family duties. However, rest does not mean just lying down in the bed. It is always better to get up and move around on your own soon after delivery. This will improve your bladder and bowel activity and reduce the risk of developing blood clots in the lower extremities. Continue taking your prenatal calcium and vitamins with iron.

In Indian culture, ghee is a must and the most important ingredient post-delivery. Our mothers and grandmothers use lots of ghee in each and every preparation (laddu, snacks, roti) for a new mother. Moderate amount of cow ghee is beneficial during your healing phase. It gives you strength, helps in smooth bowel movement, and repairs the muscles, which have gone through a lot of stress during labour. But eating a lot of ghee could play havoc with your digestive system and end up adding to your weight.

Gondh (edible gum) is considered a warming and laxative food, which is rich in calcium, potassium, and dietary fibres. During the postpartum period, it helps in the healing process. You can use gondh in making sweets dishes. Apart from this, you can continue with your pregnancy diet chart and take wholesome meals with no restriction except oil and spices.

POSTNATAL EXERCISES

Looking after your tiny toy is the best exercise that will help you in your weight-loss program. The aim of postnatal exercise is not only losing your weight, but exercise will also help you to restore the abdominal muscle tone and strength.

Good back care and posture are important because the physiological ligamentous changes during pregnancy take up to 4–5 months to reverse. Simple exercises such as pelvic tilting in different positions and alternative resting postures together with suggestions for good feeding positions, nappy changing, and baby-carrying habits may go a long way towards solving your back problems. Further, exercise makes you feel good about yourself, enhances the recovery, and provides you more energy and stamina.

Initial postnatal exercise can be started within couple of days after any kind of delivery. The first 6 weeks after delivery are crucial. Your main aim of exercise during this phase is to realign your spine and strengthen your pelvic floor muscles.

1. Deep breathing exercise is very beneficial for its circulatory and relaxing effects. Abdominal breathing or belly breathing is a wonderful abdominal tightening exercise. (Refer fig. 4.1.)

2. Kegel exercise: The importance of pelvic floor exercise after delivery is as vital as it was during pregnancy. Vagina and perineal muscles are stretched and weakened by the birth process. Kegel exercise is valuable for the toning, strengthening, and healing of these muscles. They increase the circulation of the area and thus reduce the inflammation and oedema. Pelvic floor exercise strengthens the bladder control as well. You can do it in lying, sitting, or standing position and during breastfeeding too. Do at least 50–100 contractions per day holding for 5 seconds each time. Make this exercise a habit for life; perhaps do them whenever you watch TV, while talking on

the phone, or working in the kitchen. If you have a weak bladder, the symptoms may be the following:

   a) Leaking of urine or lack of control of urine or stool.

   b) Leaking happens when you put an increased pressure on your bladder like when you cough, sneeze, or exercise.

   c) Leaking may be a small amount or less. A large amount requires a pad.

   d) If leaking is associated with pain or burning sensations while emptying the bladder, contact your doctor because you may have a bladder infection or urinary retention.

3. Walking: As early as you feel better, start with the short walks of about 5 minutes, put up to 15–20 minutes. Never exhaust yourself and follow what your body is telling you.

4. Shoulder and arm exercise: Shoulder shrugs, elbow circling, neck movements are helpful in alleviating any stiffness in your shoulder and neck joints. Arm stretching exercise and shoulder retraction will tone up your breast muscles and prevent them from sagging.

5. Join both the hands in front of your chest. Now press them hard against each other. Hold the press for few seconds and then release. Repeat this for 8–10 times. It makes your breast muscles to contract and make them tight.

6. Leg exercise: Foot and ankle stretching exercises will help in improving circulation.

After 6–8 Weeks

Now you can start all the exercises you were doing in your pregnancy. Work more on your back and abdominal muscles to regain the tone and strength. Begin your exercise steadily. Do a little warm-up like brisk walking, shoulder shrugs, neck movements, finger and wrist movements. While exercising, if you feel pain or discomfort, decrease the effort you are putting or choose a gentle form of exercise. It is always better to start your postnatal exercise program under a physiotherapist's guidance.

1. **Gentle back stretch and twist:** Lie on your back. Keeping your right leg extended, bend your left knee. Inhale and raise your right arm over your head. Exhale and feel the stretch over your right side.

   Now, cross your left leg over your right knee. Press the left foot firmly on the floor. Keep breathing normally and maintain this stretch and twist for few seconds. Exhale deeply and relax yourself. Repeat the same on the other side.

2. **Towel pulse (modified abdominal crunches):** Lie down on your back. Both the legs should be bent from the knees. Now place a towel across your upper shin (just below the knee) and hold each end. Take a deep inhalation followed by exhalation, tuck your abdominals in, and lift your head and shoulders off the floor. Pull both the ends of towel to hold the position. Release and repeat for 8–10 times initially. You can gradually increase the repetition depending

on your strength. Regular crunches will put your abdominal muscles back to shape.

Once you are able to do it comfortably, leave the towel and put your hands over your front thighs. Now lift your head and shoulders off the ground. It is very important not to lift your entire back off the floor, as this may cause back strain. (Fig. 7.1).

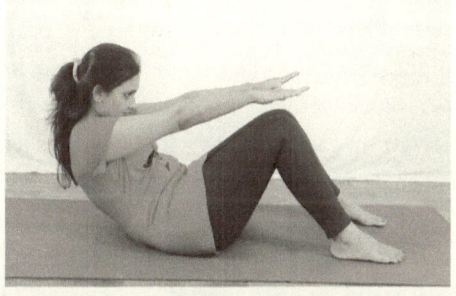

3. **Prone leg lift (Salabhasana):** Lie on your tummy. Stretch both arms up above your head. Now lift your alternate legs up from the hip joint without bending the knees. Hold each leg up for 3–4 seconds. Once you can do it comfortably, move yourself to an advanced step.

   Now, lift both the legs and both the arms up at the same time. Raise your head up. Hold this position for 3 seconds and then put all the limbs down. Keep your breathing normal. Repeat this asana for 5–6 times.

   Variation (diagonal stretch): Only in prone lying position, lift your right leg and left arm simultaneously. Hold it for a few seconds and relax.

Then lift your left leg and right arm. Continue the sequence for 6–8 times.

These exercises strengthen your abdominals, lower back, and hip muscles. They also work on your thigh muscles and reduce the flabbiness.

4. **Supine leg curls (knee to chest):** Lie on your back. Bend both the knees and bring them towards your chest. Place your hands around the back of your thighs. Stretch a little more with your hands and feel your lower back opened and released.
   Variation: Lie on your back. Bring your left leg into the chest and hug round the back of the left thigh. Allow your right leg to long down the mat. Keep your right knee completely straight. Feel the lower back and right knee opened and released. Hold it for couple of breaths and then release the left leg. Now repeat the same with the right leg. Keep breathing normally throughout.

   This exercise lengthens and stretches the lower back and thus helps to relieve back pain. Your abdominals and pelvic floor muscles also come in action.

5. **Adhomukhswanasana (down dog pose):** Come on to your hands and knees as you do in 'cat and camel' pose (all four positions). Your hands should be shoulder width apart and knees are hip width apart. Hands are in line with shoulders and knees slightly behind your hips so that you get maximum length in torso and spine when you move into Adhomukhswanasana. Press your hands firmly on

the mat and curl your toes in. Now slowly lift your knees off the floor. Stretch your arms to lengthen the torso. As you align your feet and stretch your back fully in dog pose, straighten your knees and legs as much as you can. Avoid turning your knees out. Here, the base of the spine is the apex of the pose as you stretch from the hands to the back and from your feet up your legs (Fig. 7.2).

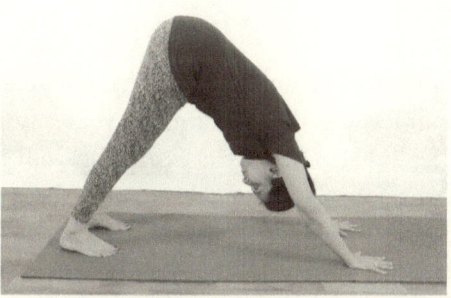

This exercise removes your fatigue and energises your body as it brings ample blood supply to the brain. It strengthens the arm muscles and removes excess fat around the waist. This brings good shape to the legs. It also relieves lower back tension and stretches hamstrings, shoulder, and spinal muscles.

Variation: Stable yourself in the dog pose. Now extend your right leg out behind you and keep your left leg slightly bent. Then lower the right leg and repeat on the other leg. Now come onto your toes and continue stretching your back as you walk your feet one by one slowly towards your hands. Keep your head relaxed and breathe normally.

6. **Buttock walk:** Sit at one corner of your room with your legs straight. Keep your hands on the thighs. Now lift your buttocks one by one and move forward as if you are moving with your hips. Move forward and reach to the other end of the room. Now without changing your position, go backwards with buttocks lift. Try to keep your knees straight. Practice 2 sets of forward and backwards moves daily. This will burn your fat around the hips and buttocks.

7. **Boat pose (Naukasana):** Lie on your back with your feet together and arms on your side. Take one deep inhalation. As you exhale, lift your chest and feet off the floor. Extend your arms forward in line with your shoulders. Balance on your sit bones by keeping your spine erect. You will feel a good contraction in your abdominal muscles. Keep breathing normally and hold the pose if you can. Come back to the floor slowly and take a relaxing breath (Fig. 7.3). Boat pose is one of the best yoga poses for core strength. It strengthens the 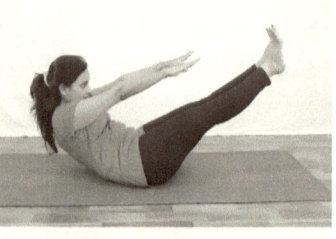 spine and abdominal muscles. It tones up your legs and abdominals. This asana builds your overall strength and power.

8. **Relaxation poses (upside down):** In yoga, it is called 'Viparita karni'. Place a folded blanket or mat

near to wall. Sit facing a wall with your buttocks about 6–8 inches away from the wall. Now lie down on your back and extend your legs up towards the ceiling. Adjust your hips and rest your buttocks and lower back on the blanket/mat.

You can hold your baby on your abdomen in the hug position. Or extend your arms by your side palms facing upward (Refer fig. 1.1). Close your eyes and relax completely for a few minutes. Continue to breathe deeply as you focus your awareness on the chest and upper back–abdomen and lower back. To come back, place feet on wall, slide buttocks off the blanket, roll onto one side, and slowly sit up. This relaxation pose induces a deep rest with the positive effects on the endocrine and nervous system. It will rapidly recharge and refresh you.

Do not go for the high-intensity aerobics or running for initial 5–6 months, because your muscles and joints are still not fully recovered from the pregnancy and childbirth effect. Swimming should be done only after your post-delivery bleeding (lochia) has been stopped.

POSTNATAL BLUES / POSTPARTUM ANXIETY / DEPRESSION

A new mother goes through a variety of good and bad emotions including joy, bliss, sometimes anger, and irritation. The common manifestations of postnatal mood swings or depressive illness vary in their time of onset and in their degree of severity. During the postpartum period, about 80% of women experience some type of mood disturbances. Among them, 15% women develop more significant symptoms of psychiatric illness.

In the initial days or weeks, mother may feel irritable, sad, weepy, and anxious. This temporary phase of mood swings is very common in many of the mothers, which is known as the 'baby blue' or 'postpartum blue'. Sometimes lack of family support, fatigue, hormonal changes, sore breasts or perineum, breastfeeding difficulties may trigger your emotional instability. This is the time you have to take very good care of yourself. Talk and discuss with your husband, friend/family, take help from others, exercise, meditate, eat well, rest, and avoid unlikely visitors. You have to reassure yourself that 'maternity blue' or depression is not your weakness or debility, it's simply a complication of giving birth. Generally, this temporary phase of maternity blue will resolve within 2–3 weeks after birth.

Research suggests that about 25% of mothers experiencing severe postnatal blues will go on to develop postnatal depression. In this depressive phase:

- You start getting the feeling of isolation, guilt, or worthlessness.
- Your concentration and energy level become low.
- You find problems in taking care of yourself and your baby. Relationship with your husband may get disturbed.
- Sleeping and eating pattern get haywire.
- Lose the interest in usual routine activities.
- Become hopeless, more apprehensive, and pessimist.

- Physical symptoms such as loss of hair and non-dietary weight gain may also be present.

Sometimes you feel so bad and ashamed of yourself that you are not enjoying the happiest time of your life. If you feel you are unable to cope up with this problem, talk to your doctor and get counselling from a mental health professional. Medications may be required to make you feel better. Along with that, you need to focus on yourself. Join a kind of postnatal classes in your area where you get chance to meet so many new mothers. Meditation, relaxation, and exercises are the remedies to stabilise your emotions, difficult thoughts, and relationships.

8

Breastfeeding – An Ultimate Experience

We women are just wondrous. We nurture a new life within us for 9 months, bring it to this amazing world, and then nurture it with the best food of the world—milk. If you have decided to breastfeed your baby, remind yourself that you are giving your baby the best start in its life. Giving your milk can be as simple as giving your love.

Just because it's natural does not mean it comes naturally or that it's easy. It can be exhausting and painful if you get it wrong. First few days and weeks of breastfeeding can be most challenging, as you and your baby both are learning this new skill together. Knowing how to prepare the breast for breastfeeding, both prior to delivery and in the early days of nursing, will help you make your nursing experience the most pleasant one.

The breast is perfectly designed for feeding. It prepares itself for feeding from the initial months of pregnancy. The blood supply to the breast and overall size of the breast increases, which leads to tingling nipples and tenderness. However, the breast size has nothing to do with how much milk your body can produce. Mother with the small breasts can feed her baby adequately and satisfactory. The tiny bumps on the areola (dark circles around the nipple) secretes a lubricant that keeps the tissues soft and bacteria free. There is no need to clean the secretion as it protects the nipple from infection.

For a healthy breastfeeding experience and to preserve the shape of your breasts, you need to take care of it right from the start of your pregnancy.

- Always wear well-fitted and cotton brassiere to support the breast. Nursing or maternity bra makes feeding easier and also prevents the breast from sagging. Avoid underwired and very tight-fitted bra as it may put pressure on the milk ducts which carry milk and will block them.
- Do not use soap to clean the nipple and areola as it will make them dry and sore. Never rub the nipple with towel.
- Expose the nipples and breasts to air daily for some time. Do not let the nipple remain moist for a long time as this will lead to cracking and infection.
- Pectoral muscles (which support the breast) exercise is very important to prevent the sagging. Always

wear well-fitted bra during exercise. Not wearing bra during exercising further spoil the shape of the bust line. However, you can remove bra during night-time.

- Use soft breast pads inside the nursing bra to soak the excessive milk secretion which may occur due to milk let-down reflex. It is important to keep you hygienic and fresh and to prevent any embarrassing incident.

- It is good idea to check for flat or inverted nipples while you are pregnant as this can make it difficult for the baby to latch on to the nipple properly. Stretching the tissues of the nipple several times a day during last months of pregnancy may help correct the flat/inverted nipple. Learn the Hoffman's technique from your doctor or antenatal therapist, which involves pulling, twisting, and rolling the nipples between your forefingers and thumbs. But sometimes this kind of nipple manipulation may cause uterine stimulation and contractions and can cause premature labour in women at risk. If it happens, discontinue nipple stretching.

Benefits of Breast Milk for Your Baby

- The American Academy of Paediatrics (AAP) says that breast milk promotes baby's healthier growth and brain development.

- Breast milk is a perfectly watched nutrition. It has almost 400 nutrients (protein, fat, carbohydrate, vitamins, minerals, and hormones), not present in any other infant food. It also changes according to the needs of your baby.

- It is easily digested by babies, so they have less stomach upset, diarrhoea, and colic (gas) trouble than do formula fed babies.
- Babies receive antibodies from their mothers against a variety of illness.
- Since there is no foreign protein in mother's milk, allergy to mother's milk does not occur.
- Studies revealed that, in the long run, your breastfed baby will be more intelligent. It has lower risk of having obesity, respiratory problems, skin problems, allergies, anaemia, heart problem, diabetes, etc.
- Baby feels love and security. Your natural body odour plays an important role in your bonding with baby. The oil released by areolas which lubricates your nipples also smells of amniotic fluid. This is familiar and attractive smell for the baby, especially right after the birth. So avoid using scented soaps, perfumes, and body lotion in the initial days particularly around the breasts.

Benefits of Breastfeeding for You

- It is very economical. You can give according to your baby's requirement. It is at proper temperature and no need to sterilize it. On the other hand, the cost of formula or infant food is very much high.
- To breastfeed your baby is very convenient for you. You can feed him anytime and anywhere.
- Breastfeeding stimulates the hormone oxytocin, which helps in shrinking off the size of the uterus and thus will help you lose some of your pregnancy weight. Breastfeeding mothers tend to have an

earlier return to their pre-pregnant weight compared with the formula-feeding moms.

- Breastfeeding your baby gives you the feeling of satisfaction and fulfilment. The hormone oxytocin promotes a strong sense of love, attachment, and closer relationship between the two of you.

- It gives you improved blood sugar control and good cholesterol profile means lower the risk of heart problems. It reduces the risk of breast/ovarian/cervical cancer as much as by 20%. It minimises the chances of suffering from postnatal depression and even post-menopausal osteoporosis (body absorbs calcium much more efficiently in pregnant and lactating mothers). The longer you breastfeed, the greater the protection.

- Research shows that breastfeeding women sleep an average of 45 minutes a night more than mothers who formula-feed and thus they report feeling less tired. This is because the sleep-inducing hormone prolactin helps you get more rest. Second, you don't have to get up from bed to prepare or warm a bottle of formula for baby.

Diet for the Lactating Mothers

After your delivery, your body experiences lots of hormonal and physical changes. Your body undergoes healing process, so you require more nutritive food to regain strength and to make more milk for your baby. Plan the best diet chart with the combination of traditional and modern way. There are some traditional galactagogue foods for milk production.

- Almond milk and date milkshake
- Pomegranate juice
- Sesame seed, flax seeds, fresh coconut, poppy seeds, dill seeds (suva), fenugreek seeds
- Finger millet (raagi), white millet (bajra), sorghum (jowar), wheat roti/bread, oat porridge

In India, some Ayurvedic medicines like Dashmoolarishta and Shatavari (asparagus) are advisable for the initial couple of months. It helps to relieve pain and inflammation. It also boosts your immunity and fastens your recovery.

The UNICEF, the World Health Organisation (WHO), American Academy of Paediatrics, and Breastfeeding Promotion Network of India (BPNI) recommend exclusive breastfeeding for the first 6 months of life and should be continued up to 2 years with adequate complementary foods. This is the best feeding strategy for infants and young children. Breastfeeding should be started as soon as possible after birth, preferably within 2 hours. This will reduce the maternal bleeding and stimulate more milk production.

The first few days after the birth, your breasts make an ideal 'first milk' called 'colostrums'. It is thick yellowish fluid with the perfect combination of nutrients and antibodies and thus builds up baby's immunity. Colostrums are high in protein, less in fat and sugar, and very easily digested by baby, so consider it as a liquid gold for your baby. It helps newborn's digestive tract to develop and prepare itself to digest breast milk. Usually babies will lose 5–8% weight in the first 3–5 days of birth due to the fluid loss and extra fat loss. So the weight loss is not related to breastfeeding. Just don't start top (formula) feed for your baby in a hurry.

A healthy baby regains its birth weight again within 10–12 days. And after that, if your baby gains approximately 150 g of weight per week (20 g/day) and if baby passes urine 10–12 times/day and 3–5 bowel movements/day means, he is getting sufficient breast milk for his normal growth.

After a few days of birth, your body will make more mature milk. Each time you feed your baby, milk changes throughout the feeding session. The initial milk baby gets (foremilk) is watery, mild bluish, and containing lactose, which satisfy baby's thirst. So baby does not require outside water even in hot, summer season. The hind milk is creamier, thick, and containing fat to satisfy baby's hunger and is the main source of energy for your baby. Make sure your baby feeds for longer time to one breast (approximate 10–15 minutes) so he can get benefits of hind milk also. Always remind yourself that you have to feed your baby from both breasts equally. If your baby falls asleep or refuse for the feed before you've switched breast, next time you offer him the missed breast first. Your body will over time adjust and produce only the amount of milk your baby needs. The flavour of the breast milk changes according to your diet means your baby is already acquiring different tastes. You can feed your baby even if you or your baby is sick. In some cases where mother has hepatitis, infectious disease, had some breast surgery, or mother is taking drugs for cancer/seizure, breastfeeding is not recommended.

Preparation and Positioning

Your baby is smart enough to give you some hints that he is hungry now. Look for the signs like hands in mouth, moving head side to side, sucking objects, rapid eye movement or stirring, which indicate hunger. Nurse your baby before he starts crying.

Whenever you take your baby to feed, first prepare yourself by washing your hands and take a comfortable position. You will have to sit upright while nursing your baby. You can use proper-sized nursing (feeding) pillow or a number of regular pillows for comfort of your baby and your back. Breastfeeding makes you very much thirsty, so always take a glass of water beside you while you feed.

It is proven that relaxed mother can produce more milk and satisfy her baby. Stress level can affect the quantity of milk. So if you are tensed, take a few deep breaths and relax your body and mind. Even between the feeding sessions, you can lie down for relaxation and meditate.

Align your baby so that he/she is tummy to tummy with you. You can use pillow/s in your lap to take the baby at your breast level. Baby's face and body both should be completely turned towards you (bring your baby to your breast, not your breast to your baby). Support the baby's head and neck with one hand. With the other hand, hold your breast in 'C' hold and gently lift and support it. Make sure your fingers are well away from the areolar tissues.

Now, gently stroke the baby's lower lip with your nipple to exhibit the rooting reflex. Make sure his mouth is wide enough to take in nipple, areola, and somewhat breast tissues as well. This is called proper 'latch on'. If baby sucks on the nipple only, it results in inadequate milk, so the vigorously hungry baby bites on nipple to get more milk.

This makes your nipple sore and cracked, which will be a painful situation. Milk will be secreted adequately only if baby suckles well on areola (Fig. 8.1).

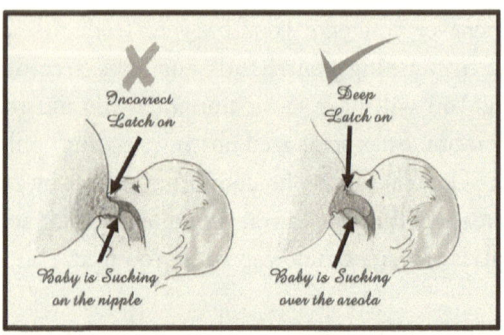

Signs of Good Latch On

If your baby is latched on correctly, both his lips will pout (upper lip will bend upwards and lower lip roll back towards the chin). His tongue is over lower gum and muscles below the ears move as he sucks and swallows. If your baby sucks noisily and gets hungry very frequently or you get hurt/uncomfortable during feeding, that means baby doesn't latch on perfectly. A typical rhythm of breastfeeding—suck, swallow, and breathe; again suck, swallow, and breathe— is well developed in full-term babies. Babies need your complete attention, so maintain eye contact, talk to him, or sing rhymes/lullabies while nursing. Watching television, talking to someone else on phone while feeding will never satisfy your baby.

Just like latch on, proper latch off is very important to avoid sore nipples. To take baby off the breast, slide your little finger into the corner of baby's mouth. As baby opens the mouth little wide, break the suction.

After each feed, clean your nipples with plain water and dry them naturally. Vigorous rubbing will lose their moisture and make them cracked. Once your baby is done with feeding, hold him erect over your shoulder or make him sit straight in your lap (in both position, support the baby's head to prevent it from dropping). Now, pat or rub its back gently so that the swallowed air is let out by burping. 'Burping' is very important after every feeding session, or baby will suffer from the colic (gas) pain. Sometimes it may happen that after several minutes of patting, baby may not eruct. Some babies may take out some amount of milk after feeding, which is normal. But repeated vomiting should not be neglected.

For the first month of birth, your newborn should be nursed 8–12 times a day. Frequent feeding will stimulate your milk production during initial weeks. Then gradually baby will be fed 7–9 times a day. Newborn should not go more than 4 hours without feeding even at night-time. Once your milk supply is established and your baby is a little mature now, feeding on demand (when baby is hungry) is the best idea rather than a fixed schedule. Time spent in sucking varies between 10 and 30 minutes.

Thoughts of a baby, smell of baby or baby products, baby crying sound, or just seeing other babies may lead to let-down reflex (automatic release of breast milk). You can express (take out) your breast milk either manually or with the breast pump and store it when you are going to separate from your baby for long hours. So your partner or caregiver can feed your baby your milk from a bottle or a sipper. Electric breast pump is an easier and quicker way to express milk. Choosing the right pump and using it properly is a key to maintaining your milk supply.

For storage of milk, always use a sterilised bottle and label it with the time you store it. Breast milk can sustain its nutrients for up to 3 hours in an open (room temperature), 2–3 days in refrigerator (4°C), and for about 4 months in the deep freezer. Never boil or defrost breast milk by putting it in the microwave oven or on gas stove. This kind of heating process will destroy the antibodies and can change the composition of milk. Bring the milk to room temperature indirectly by putting the bottle/cup in the warm water. Once defrosted and used, milk should not be put back in the fridge and you need to discard it.

Breastfeeding Issues

It may happen that due to lack of awareness and knowledge, many women experience the breastfeeding as a terrible task. In the initial months only, they have to introduce formula milk and stop breastfeeding their babies because of some of the following factors.

1. **Insufficient milk supply:** Milk production is a demand and supply process. If you have any doubts and you are concerned about your milk supply, you can meet a breastfeeding counsellor or a certified lactation consultant. Sometimes fatigue, anxiety, stress, poor diet, or excessive consumption of caffeine can reduce milk supply. To increase the production of milk, do the following:

- **Nurse your baby frequently** and for a long time. Offer both breasts in each feeding session.
- **Take enough rest.** An exhausted underfed mother is not an efficient milk producer. Eat well-balanced diet and take sufficient amount of liquids. You will need to consume extra 500 calories more per day than before pregnancy. You should continue your prenatal vitamin to meet your body's increased needs.
- Use '**galactagogues**' (substances that increase the milk supply). Some household herbal galactagogues are fenugreek seeds, coconut, sesame seeds, whole grains especially oat meal, nuts especially almonds, cumin seeds, anise seeds, fennel seeds, carom, black sesame seeds, flax seeds, etc. There are several prescribed medications also that can improve your milk supply.

2. **Engorgement:** Your breasts become heavy and full of milk if baby has not been fed for a long time. Sometimes your breasts become hard, tender, and swollen. This condition is very uncomfortable and painful for you and difficult for the baby to latch on properly. To avoid engorgement, breastfeed your baby frequently or take out milk manually or with breast pump as soon as you start feeling heaviness. Use alternate breast for feeding every time.

   For the relief from pain and swelling, use cold packs or warm shower bath between the feeds. Gentle massage (downward strokes towards nipple) to your breasts before feeding will soften the areola and baby can latch on easily. Compressing strokes help drain the breast, leaving less milk behind.

3. **Sore and cracked nipple:** Nipple soreness usually occurs in the initial weeks of nursing. If you continue to feed your baby in an incorrect position, the soreness will increase and nipple may crack, become red and bleed. Nipple pain becomes so severe that you dread putting your baby to your breasts.

- To prevent the occurrence, make sure that baby takes whole nipple and areola in the mouth and latches on and off to your breast properly. As we discussed earlier, don't use soap or any lotion to your breasts. Expose nipple to air-dry after feedings. Always wear cotton and slightly loose bra and use good quality breast pads/cloth inside it.

- Unfortunately if soreness and cracks appear, you can apply ice pack to sore nipple before feeding for the pain relief and soothing effect. Change the feeding positions every time, e.g., try sitting, lying, cradle or football hold position so that the pressure from the baby's sucking will not be in the same place all the time. Apply your hind milk on the affected nipple for healing which has an excellent anti-infective property.

- Baby should be offered the least sore breast first. In case of a severe problem, use a thin silicon 'nipple shield', which is easily available in the market. It is the flexible nipple-shaped silicon that should be worn directly over your nipple during feeding. Even if you have flat, inverted, or poorly formed nipple, you can still breastfeed your baby with the use of nipple puller. Nipple puller is convenient and safe, which can help to draw out inverted nipples. Gentle massage to the breasts help to open mammary glands and thus enable breastfeeding.

4. **Blocked ducts:** Sometimes milk tubes get blocked because of wearing tight bra or some other reason and milk starts accumulating behind the blockage which will ultimately result in the formation of lump (a painful, hard, and red patch). The pain can be reduced by applying hot fomentation or cold compresses. Keep offering your baby the affected breast first and massage the lump towards the nipple as you feed. This will help to unblock the duct. Keep on changing your feeding positions (cradle, football, and crossover) so that all the milk ducts get stimulated equally. Consult your doctor if it is not getting clear, because it can lead to mastitis (a bacterial infection) if not taken care properly.

5. **Mastitis:** This is not a very common problem, but still all breastfeeding mothers should have a little idea about it. Mastitis is an inflammation in the breast tissues due to insufficient drainage of the breast (milk stasis). In some countries, it is also called as 'milk fever'. You need to take an antibiotic course. Continue feeding may help treat the mastitis. Don't worry; this infection does not affect the quality of breast milk. In contrast, stopping the breastfeeding will make the condition worse.

Fever, pain, and swelling will make you a little down, but try to take enough rest and drink plenty of fluids. Do some arm encircling exercises (without wearing a bra) to unclog the ducts and for strengthening. If you have abscess in one of the breasts, continue feeding your baby with the other breast. But remember to empty your mastitis breast frequently.

6. **Thrush (rare problem):** It is a kind of fungal infection, which may affect both mother and baby. It can trigger a sharp stabbing pain, which radiates deep into the breast. Your nipples become pink/red, itchy, shiny, and burning. Your baby may have white patch on its tongue or mouth. You both need treatment for it. You can ask your doctor about the effects of drugs on the breast milk and, in turn, the baby. However, common analgesics like NSAIDs are considered to be safe with breastfeeding. Very small amounts do end up in the breast milk, but this amount is quite less to have any effect on your newborn.

Fathers can be an important side of breastfeeding triangle (mom, dad and baby) to make it the successful one. However, you are not directly involved in the process, but your understanding, encouragement, and positive support is the most valuable help to your wife and baby, especially in the initial weeks, when lack of sleep and hormonal changes make the new mother more frustrated and anxious. Over that time, it will be a great help if you can burp the baby or can change his nappies. Baby needs lots of physical contact, so when not breastfeeding, father's loving arms are the most wonderful place for a baby. As much more time you spend with your baby, it will be turned in a strong bond with your baby.

If you want to get in touch with other breastfeeding mothers or seek more guidance and information about all the aspect of breastfeeding, you can search for the Mother's Support Group (MSG) in your area or can contact 'La Leche League' (International Organisation on Breastfeeding) in your city.

9

Myths And Beliefs Of Pregnancy

Pregnancy is a universal phenomenon, so every place in the world has its own share of beliefs and myths about pregnancy. In India, we have a large social crowd around us ready to give us so many advices and suggestions for baby's well-being. For example, your grandmother might have told you to not take tea in pregnancy or else your baby's complexion will be dark, rather drink saffron milk to get a fair-skinned baby. If you drink coconut water, your baby will have lot of hair on his/her body. Your elderly neighbour may tell you that pregnant women should not eat papaya; it can cause miscarriage. If you are suffering from morning sickness, you are going to deliver a girl child. And so the list goes on. After getting different advices and beliefs from different people, you become confused and sometimes stressed that what to believe and what to do for a smooth and healthy pregnancy. But don't worry. You need to understand your body, your pregnancy, and just follow your doctor's guidance. Here, we will discuss some of the very common myths or beliefs of pregnancy and labour.

1. **Prediction about baby's sex:** It's a usual belief that if you have got a high belly, you are expecting a baby girl, and if you are carrying your baby low, you will have a boy. Baby's sex can't be determined by how high or low you are carrying a child. How you carry a baby is determined by your baby's size and position, your body type, and muscular tone of the womb.

   It is a usual myth that if pregnant lady is craving for salty food, she is most likely to deliver a baby boy, and if she is craving for sweets, she will deliver a girl child. But the fact is that craving is a result of your hormonal changes. Sometimes it depends on your body needs and deficiency of nutrients like calcium or iron. If you have strong cravings for non-food items like chalk or crayons, then your body might be lacking in calcium.

2. **You should eat for two:** Practically, no one can eat for two people at a time. If she is forced to eat for two, amount of weight she puts on will be hard to lose after baby's birth. Sometimes excess weight can lead to more serious consequences. Your baby is a parasite and completely depends on you, so you should choose the stuff that does not increase your fat, but at the same time provides proper nutrition for the baby's growth. Pregnancy is not about eating for two, but eating a well-balanced

diet. In pregnancy, you need only 350 extra calories per day, so it implies that you should eat about one and a fifth. This is equal to a normal diet plus 24 almonds or 2 eggs.

3. **Sexual intercourse will hurt my baby:** Baby is actually protected by the cushioning effects of amniotic fluid. Even there is a safety seal called mucus plug on the cervix. In addition, there are 7 layers of skin, muscles, tissue, and fat from the abdominal wall to the amniotic sac, so baby is fully protected and safe. A pregnant woman can have sexual relations as long as she is comfortable.

   Still it is advisable not to have sex in first and 3rd trimester, especially for the women at high risk of miscarriage (if you have one or more miscarriages before). Even if you have any pain, staining (red discharge), or uneasiness after intercourse, stop having sex. In the 1st trimester, you may not have great desire for sex due to sickness and fatigue. In the 3rd trimester, you are not comfortable with your overly rounded tummy.

4. **If pregnant mother has swelling over her face and extremities, she should drink very less water:** False. As your uterus is growing, it puts pressure on your pelvic veins and the vena cava (the large vein that carries blood from the lower limbs to the heart). This pressure slows down the return of blood from the legs, and blood gets collected there. This leads to swelling of the ankles and feet. Sometimes swelling over hands and face is the result of increased body fluid and retention of water.

Don't cut down your water intake. You need to drink at least 8-10 glasses of water daily in order to get rid your system of excess sodium and other waste products. This will ultimately reduce the swelling. Limit your salt intake will be beneficial.

5. **Sitting down on the floor will give rise to premature delivery:** Squatting for a long time in the 1st trimester is not advisable. But sitting cross-legged on the floor is absolutely harmless. Rather, tailor sitting (cross-legged sitting) is especially recommended in the last trimester to reduce the lower back pain and to increase the flexibility of the pelvic joints. So that at the time of delivery, pelvic opens up easily. (This is the reason why sweeper ladies get very easy delivery.)

6. **Umbilical cord is attached with mother's umbilicus:** This is a false belief. Many pregnant women don't have any idea about this. Actually, one end of umbilical cord is attached with placenta (a part of uterus) and the other end is attached with baby's umbilicus. Umbilical cord and placenta are the part of foetal life support system. Placenta prepares food and nutrition for the baby and it reaches to the baby via the umbilical cord. After baby's birth, placenta should be removed and umbilical cord will be clamped.

7. **Eat one spoon ghee or castor oil every day in the last months for easy delivery:** Our grandmothers believe that castor oil or ghee lubricates the birth canal (vagina) and make it more slippery and smooth, so

baby can easily be delivered. This is completely wrong concept. However, castor oil may induce labour in some cases. It is a powerful laxative which tends to irritate the intestine and cause loose motion. As the nerve supply to the intestine and the uterus is the same, uterine contractions get initiated. But castor oil has very unpleasant side effect of nausea and diarrhoea. It is not at all recommended nowadays.

To make your labour and delivery easy, you need to do exercises and breathing. Exercise proves to be more helpful in increasing the flexibility of the pelvic area. Cow ghee has many good properties—it is high in unsaturated fat so it should be consumed moderately. Otherwise it will just add fat in your body and accelerate weight gain. In ancient times, ladies were engaged in many physical work, they did many households work by themselves, so they could easily digest ghee.

8. **Labour is a very painful process:** Labour is a natural process in which uterus contracts and tries to push the baby out. So of course labour is painful, but not up to the extent that you can't cope up. Pain threshold varies individually. Each woman has a different pain tolerance level. Stress and fear will increase your pain and discomforts, but your confidence and positive attitude along with the breathing exercise will definitely ease your labour and delivery. In our body, when we get extreme pain that we can't bear, we become unconscious as we see in many road accidents or so. But during labour, no woman has gone unconscious. If you know the proper techniques of breathing at proper

time of labour contractions, you can easily cope up with your pain.

Nowadays if you are not coping up with the pain, you can opt for epidural anaesthesia (painless labour).

9. **Push your baby down while you are in labour pain:** This is a wrong conviction. Don't push until your doctor says so. If you are in the early or intermediate phase of labour, then your cervix is not completely dilated, i.e., 10 cm. If you push during that time, baby's head will hit to the non-dilated cervix, which is dangerous for the baby. Even this will cause pain and swelling of your cervix too. If you have urge to push, but you are not fully dilated, just hold back and do pant-blow breathing.

10. **Abdominal belt flattens the tummy post-delivery:** You can use abdominal belt for initial 3–4 weeks. It will provide good support to your stretched and flabby muscles. It also supports your back muscles and spinal cord and thus relieves your back pain. It keeps your body erect and improves your posture.

But abdominal belt solely is not very effective. You can forcefully tighten your muscles with belt, but next time when you take out the belt, your muscles will be as it is. Sometimes too much tight belt exerts much pressure on the uterus and can cause bleeding. Even many women find it uncomfortable, painful, and inconvenient. So better you do exercise and take healthy diet for a few months and come back in shape again.

11. **Read good books and be happy:** If your mother or grandmother is telling you that you should read good religious books like Bhagavad Gita, Ramayana, or Bible during pregnancy, they are very much true this time. You have to spend some time in reading quality books and listening to some devotional or instrumental music. Books and music have been seen to reduce high stress level that many women experience during their pregnancy. They will remove your unwanted thoughts and give you mental peace. Music may help in foetal brain development and also strengthens the bond with your unborn child. Avoid watching action movies and reading detective novels as this kind of input will increase your fear, anxiety, and thus indirectly affect your baby's mental and physical health.

If you are stressed or tensed, bad hormones (adrenaline) will release from your body. This is not good for you and your baby. Mom's stress during pregnancy may have long-lasting negative effects on child's behaviour, emotions, and cognitive development.

Indulge yourself in some recreational activities like art, painting, and music. Mental activities like puzzles and Sudoku will improve your baby's IQ.